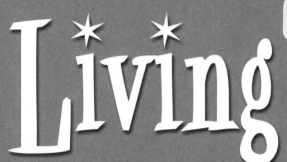

Living Sexy Fit

...at any age!

To Sarah!
Celebrating
you!
x Kate
McKay

Kate McKay

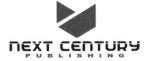

NEXT CENTURY
PUBLISHING

Living Sexy Fit!
At Any Age!

Published by Next Century Publishing
www.NextCenturyPublishing.com

ISBN: 978-162-9030555

Limit of Liability/Disclaimer of Warranty

Cover photo by JWAtherton www.jwathertonimages.com

Printed in the United States of America

www.LivingSexyFit.com

In Gratitude...

To even begin to list the people who have inspired me to live my life all out would read like *War and Peace*. However, I would like to send out my deep gratitude and appreciation to the following amazing people:

To my mom, who celebrated my living my life "too big for my britches," and to my dad, for modeling extreme self-care and a fit lifestyle, and for modeling passion and commitment to his work.

To my seven zany siblings near and far, who even through the struggles and challenges of life still live with open and kind hearts.

To my kids, Will, John, and Sophie, who know their mom is just plumb all-out crazy about life, and love me anyway. It's because of them that I am so committed to making the world a better place.

To my amazing friends, Jodie, Elaine, Jamie, Stephanie, Katie, and so many more, who keep me real and provide a level of safety and encouragement that pushes me to keep living into my life.

To the many coaches I have had, both in business and in fitness, including but not limited to Nancy McCabe, Susie Carder, Lisa Nichols, Janelle Nicolo, and Michele Scism. These women always believed in me, even when I didn't.

To my accountant Jeff Kirpas and my attorney Susan Finneran, for supporting my mission and making sure I was doing it smart and with integrity.

To the women who helped me with typing my book from my chicken-scratch notes, Emily Daniels, Sue Guido and Laura Henderson. Thank you! Also, thank you, Karen LaManuzzi for letting us use the Fitness Studio for our photo shoot.

Thank you also to Michael Mirdad, my spiritual guide and healer, who never let me wallow and always kept me centered on God and my bigger purpose.

Big kudos to my Body Ambition fitness family for creating such a wonderful place where we can celebrate our victories and challenges together. We are never alone!

And a huge thank you to my Global Leadership family and the Lisa Nichols Motivating the Masses organization. Words cannot describe the love, support, and open-heartedness that you model and share.

And finally, I would like to express my gratitude to two amazing men who no longer walk the planet but still challenge and inspire me every day: Mike Champagne, who was my trainer and dear friend. And my baby brother, Matthew McKay. Your spirit lives on, bro.

With Joy and Gratitude,

— *Kate McKay*

Say What?!

Living Sexy Fit?

What Does THAT Mean?

Sexy: fully vital, confident, passionate, and celebratory!

Fit: having a body that reflects your deep and passionate nature, living a life of health, wellness, and positive self-acceptance from the inside out.

The Living Sexy Fit Manifesto:

Living sexy "fit" means having bodies that reflects our deep and passionate natures, embracing lives of health, wellness, and positive self-acceptance from the inside out.

Living Sexy Fit!—It's Your Time!

If not you, then who?
What are you waiting for?
Are you waiting for the engraved invitation that shows you the time and place
That your true life will begin,
That wonderfully delicious place
Where crystal clear clarity and your peace and wellness reside?

Guess what?
You already have it.
It is within you.

Waiting for you to call it forth.
Embrace it,
And then run like the wind with it,
Joy-filled as all get-out!

Because it is yours,
You deserve it.
Positive self-worth and health!

And once you have it,
You want to share it,
Your well-being and joy,
With everyone.

Because you are blessed,
And you know,
Deep in your soul,
That you have a strong and willing spirit
And have what it takes
To live your
Breakthrough Life!

Let the wild rumpus start!

Table of Contents

In Gratitude… 3

Introduction 11

PART ONE: The Living Sexy Fit Lifestyle Holistic Approach 13

CHAPTER 1: The Living Sexy Fit Promise 15

CHAPTER 2: The Proof Is in the Pudding – *A Lifetime Dedicated to Fitness*..........17

CHAPTER 3: The Living Sexy Fit Lifestyle Holistic Approach....................23

    Let's Start Living Sexy Fit Here 24

    KATE'S BREAKDOWN TO BREAKTHROUGH!...........................28

PART TWO: Living Sexy Fit Motivational Mojo.................................31

CHAPTER 4: Motivational Mojo – *From the Inside Out* 33

    Internal vs. External Motivators...34

    GET REAL: FACING WHAT IS!..36

    Staying Positive in a Largely Negative World!............................39

CHAPTER 5: Motivational Mojo: Tolerations – *Giving a Boot to Your Hot Mess!*.43

    Celebrate and Radiate! 46

CHAPTER 6: Motivational Mojo – *Revisiting the Holistic Approach to Your Health and Hotness!*..49

CHAPTER 7: Motivational Mojo – *Why Living a Life of Integrity Is Sexy* 53

CHAPTER 8: Motivational Mojo: Getting Clear – *Creating Healthy Relationships with Yourself and Others* 59

CHAPTER 9: Motivational Mojo – *Action Plan to Living Sexy Fit*..........................67

Living Sexy Fit Goal Implementation! 72

Using the Power of Intention to Transform Your Life by Setting B.I.G. Goals! .73

CHAPTER 10: Motivational Mojo: Fear and Resistance – *Being Your Own Stick in the Mud and How to BREAK THROUGH Using the Power of Affirmation* 77

Fear – False Expectations Appearing Real! 79

PART THREE: The Living Sexy Fit Clean Eats Plan 83

CHAPTER 11: The Living Sexy Fit Clean Eats Mojo Revealed 85

CHAPTER 12: The Living Sexy Fit Clean Eats Lifestyle 87

CHAPTER 13: The Living Sexy Fit Clean Eats Lifestyle – *Nutritional Mojo* 93

"CAN'T I JUST DO THE TREADMILL AND BE DONE?" 93

The 80/20 Rule of the Living Sexy Fit Lifestyle 97

CHAPTER 14: The Living Sexy Fit Clean Eats System – *Choosing Foods That Fuel the Machine!* 99

Micronutrients 106

CHAPTER 15: The Living Sexy Fit Clean Eats System – *the Importance of Metabolism and Hydration!* 109

CHAPTER 16: The Living Sexy Fit Clean Eats Playbook 115

HOW TO "CHEAT" ON THE LSF PROGRAM 120

PORTION CONTROL 122

Clean Eats Food Preparation: 123

CHAPTER 17: Recipes for the Living Sexy Fit Lifestyle 127

PART FOUR: The Living Sexy Fit Buff Body Plan 139

CHAPTER 18: The Living Sexy Fit Buff Body Bootie Shake – *You Gotta' Move It, Move It!* 141

CHAPTER 19: The Living Sexy Fit Buff Body Plan.................................147

   THE FIVE COMPONENTS OF FITNESS.................................147

CHAPTER 20: The Living Sexy Fit Buff Body System 151

   Strength Training 101.................................153

   Strength Training Guidelines.................................155

CHAPTER 21: The Living Sexy Fit Buff Body Cardio System.................................159

   CARDIOVASCULAR EXERCISE – GO FOR THE GLOW!.................................159

   The Components of a Cardiovascular Work-Out 160

   Monitoring Exercise Intensity the Living Sexy Fit Way! 162

   Borg Rating of Perceived Exertion (RPE) 163

   Kate Gets Real!.................................167

CHAPTER 22: Living Sexy Fit Motivational Mojo and Exercise – *It's Not About Finding Time; It's About Making Time!* 169

CHAPTER 23: The Living Sexy Fit Exercise Program 171

   Suitcase Squats.................................173

PART FIVE: Living Sexy Fit Putting the Plan into Action 199

CHAPTER 24: Living the Sexy Fit Lifestyle – *Putting It All Together!* 201

   Vision Creation – Letting Loose Your Passion 204

   Your Personal Living Sexy Fit Goals 207

28-Day Living Sexy Fit Plan 210

The 28-Day Exercise Plan 212

FAQs 217

ABOUT KATE MCKAY© 221

REFERENCES 223

LIST OF RECOMMENDED READING 223

APPENDIX 225

My Living Sexy Fit Commitment 226

FOOD SHOPPING LIST 227

Introduction

Hello and welcome to the Living Sexy Fit Lifestyle! Here in the land of Inner Hottie Heaven, we believe that being fit and sexy starts from within.

The Living Sexy Fit Lifestyle takes a holistic approach because, as with any transformation, the rebirth begins on the inside. The LSF lifestyle incorporates a mind, body, spirit method to getting fit; you can't make changes in one area without affecting the others.

Holistic: ("holos"-whole) of or relating to the consideration of the complete person, physically and psychologically.

As your Coach and Cheering Squad, I am 100% focused on helping you, guiding you, inspiring you, and, if I have to, kicking your butt to ensure that you reach your goals. I am here to hold your vision of health and wellness for you.

If I see you lose that vision, I will do what I have to do to remind you, cajole you, humor you, and challenge you to go all out. Sometimes you won't like me. I'm okay with that.

To be perfectly honest, I will not let you settle for less than you deserve or desire. This is my commitment, and this is why my commitment to YOUR success is bar none. It's what drives me on a daily basis – to inspire you to have the courage and faith to go all out.

Kate News Flash: Within the LSF program, you have to be open to shifts in your self-perception, to be committed to release self-defeating language and behaviors, and to be ready, really ready, to live your breakthrough life.

The process is not always easy, but I promise you it will be worth it.

Will you trust me on that?

Please do not cut yourself short. I want you to succeed, and I will do all I can to ensure that your dream becomes your reality.

Beware! Watch throughout this book for **Hottie Hazards** that could impede your progress!

PART ONE

The Living Sexy Fit Lifestyle
Holistic Approach

CHAPTER 1

The Living Sexy Fit Promise

Are you ready to:

- live your life full out?
- unleash your Inner Hottie who's waiting to be re-born?
- let go of self-sabotaging behaviors and thinking that are making you live your life way too small?
- recalibrate the way you think about food so you can go back to enjoying your food
- increase your overall vitality and sex appeal?
- reclaim your inner peace and joy in living?

If you answered a wholehearted yes to the above, congratulations for putting yourself at the center of your breakthrough life!

For those of you who are just hearing about the Living Sexy Fit Lifestyle, climb aboard! We're so excited to have you as a part of this Hottie Hoedown!

The Living Sexy Fit Lifestyle is about redefining and embracing your "sexy" – that part of you that is full of vitality, confidence, passion, and celebration.

We embrace the fact that living "fit" means having bodies that reflects our deep and passionate natures. It means living lives of health, wellness, and positive self-acceptance from the inside out.

The Living Sexy Fit Lifestyle is about living a life of integrity and grace, about having a body that's a reflection of your inner peace, joy, and power. It's about turning on high the ole' self-love, because the bottom line is this: WITHOUT POSITIVE SELF-WORTH AND INNER SPICY MOJO, OUR HOTTIE AND VITALITY FACTORS FIZZLE LIKE A SPARKLER IN A RAINSTORM.

Mojo defined: "A charm or a spell. A power that seems magical and allows someone to be very effective or successful, or to have more sex appeal!"

CHAPTER 2

The Proof Is in the Pudding – *A Lifetime Dedicated to Fitness*

I remember the first time I held a weight in my hand. I was a junior at Bennington College – a misfit Irish Catholic Bostonian in a predominantly Jewish New York school. Clove cigarette filled the air, and the preferred wardrobe was black. The incongruity of the beautiful pastoral setting of the Bennington campus and the school's teeming punk rock kids from Long Island was both humorous and unnerving.

Frankly, the only way I was able to differentiate myself at a school like this, where I was on a full scholarship – the token poor kid, as I often described myself – was to become a jock. In the early 1980s there was no gym facility at the school, so a few of us teamed together, got hold of some old weight equipment, and converted a small space behind the mailroom into a makeshift gym.

The equipment was old and rusty. I remember lying back on the bench press. As I lifted the weight up off the rack, I had a sensation similar to the hours I spent on my hands as a child. The weight felt good, like a stretch and pressure to the system, and it somehow calmed me, making me feel centered and peaceful. I sat up after my first set feeling dizzy. From that first set, you could say I was hooked!

After I graduated from Bennington in 1985, I moved back to Boston and became part of the fitness craze of the '80s. I cut my T-shirts way before *Flash Dance* – by the time the movie came out, the Jennifer Beal look was passé. I belonged to a gym called Women's World, hot pink and flashy. The jiggle machines – where you strapped a belt around your butt and flipped the switch and jiggled your way to fitness – were front and center when you walked into the club. The older ladies hung out there and shimmied and shook with looks of bland disconnect.

It was there that I took my first aerobics class from bleached-blonde girls with hot-pink leg warmers. One instructor reminded me of Barbie – perky, beautiful, and rail thin. We all wanted to be her. A couple of weeks after starting my workout regime at the club of hot pink, I distinctly remember sitting in a chair and placing my hands on the chair arms, lifting my legs up with the use of my newfound abs. Wow! It felt amazing!

After being at Women's World for a few months, I grew weary of the culture of the club. I visited a coed gym owned by a Russian mother and daughter. These women ran the gym like it was the Russian Union; they expected everyone to use strict form and to obey their method of exercise, or they would show you the door. It was here that I met my cute Italian boyfriend who introduced me to the world of Arnold Schwarzenegger and Rachel McLeish, the hot body builders of the '80s. My boyfriend, Joe, a Sylvester Stallone lookalike, was a dreamboat and in control. Joe went on a search to find us the perfect gym and came to me one night victorious.

Universe Gym had posters of all the past and present bodybuilders plastered on the walls. It was located on the top floor in a dirty old factory in a wasteland in Somerville, Massachusetts. We felt instantly at home. The gym was hardcore. I loved it! No air conditioning, loud music, hunky men, and, not surprisingly, no girls except for a handful of brave souls.

If you had to use the bathroom, you had to ask the owner, and one of the guys at the gym would "watch" the door while you used the men's room. They were honored to do it, standing there, ensuring my complete and utter privacy. I felt taken care of, part of a family, and learned everything I needed to know about sculpting the human form, our seemingly bizarre but completely dedicated art form.

I was busy working as a property manager and exercising and having fun. In fact, I met my husband at a gym in Boston in 1990. We married in 1994. It was a tumultuous marriage, with too many moves and job changes to count. The gym remained my sanctuary through the years, despite the chaos of my marriage.

Through the late '90s, I was busy birthing and mothering my three children. Pregnancy was not easy for me, and the morning sickness knocked me to my knees for weeks at a time. But once I birthed my first two kids, I was back at the gym and got back in shape relatively quickly despite the 30 to 35-pound pregnancy weight gain.

However, after I had my third child, a daughter, in 2001, something shifted for me and I wasn't sure what. I felt uneasy within myself. My anxiety and self-doubt reached critical mass at this time, and I knew that something seriously had to change.

One of the changes I decided to take on was to get my body back, and that meant getting my out-of-shape, mommy body to a gym, PRONTO. I hired a trainer. I found a "real gym" in Amesbury, Massachusetts, called Hard Nocks. Does the name describe it for you? Ha!

Wammo! My Own Personal Transformation.
Nothing Like Getting Hit by a Cosmic 2x4!

Have you ever had a time in your life when everything you believed to be true fell completely by the wayside? You'd look in your closet and wonder, "Who bought all these clothes?" You'd look in the mirror and ask, "Who styled this hair-do? Whose body is this?" You'd look across the breakfast table at your significant other and think, "Who are YOU?"

Well, walking into that gym was THAT time for me, and I knew that for some reason, there was no turning back! It was like everything was so crystal clear and completely unrecognizable, all at the same time! I was committed to something, and I wasn't even clear what it was, but all I knew is that there was no turning back.

Can you relate?

Personal transformation is just like that. For as much as you want to pretend that everything is just as it was, you and I both know that once you wake up, and I mean, really WAKE UP, you just can't pretend to go back to sleep, no matter how hard you try.

And I tried, let me tell you! As sick as it all is, I was *seriously, almost comically*, attached to my self-doubt and self-loathing, my less-than-stellar relationships, and my life being so wacked and out of balance.

But as Anthony Robbins describes it, oftentimes transformation doesn't happen until we **get so disturbed** with a situation that we finally cry uncle!

What will it take for you to finally take the plunge and be "all in" to the best version of you?

HOW BAD DO YOU WANT IT?

What is the number one reason why so many of us say "Never Mind" only days, sometimes moments, after committing to making a change for what is ultimately in our best interest—body, mind, and soul—to lose weight and get fit?

As a fitness coach, I continue to be surprised by how heavily the extra pounds "weigh" on the spirits of my clients, the soul-sucking defeat of not doing what you desire. And I say, "I want more for you, because I see that you want it and you are worthy of that," and I see the shift, the knowing, and the commitment is sealed – both mine and theirs.

But the fact is, in life, we need concrete steps, because, bottom line, change is 99.9% of the time a <u>SOLO MISSION</u>. You know this, and that is why you bail, jump ship, bag your weight-loss fitness mission. Because we are not conditioned to do things alone. And frankly, ALONE sucks sometimes – okay, a lot of times – when you are struggling. I know it, you know it, but sometimes you gotta do what you gotta do!

And now the BIG QUESTION for you: How bad you want it and why? If not now, when? When? When?

OK, so I get all hot under the collar when I talk about this because, heck, I want you to be in your brilliance! Nothing charges me more than to see people embrace who they truly are and who they came here to be!

I know it is hard, I really do, but it is going to be so worth it! Happy Dance!

I am so excited for you to be a part of the Living Sexy Fit journey. Let's go!

CHAPTER 3

The Living Sexy Fit Lifestyle Holistic Approach

The Living Sexy Fit Lifestyle takes a holistic approach to getting and staying fit. While eating clean and exercise are important and key elements to the plan, your inner work, or your **Motivational Mojo**, that "something" that makes you tick, is at the foundation of rocking your hotness and living the breakthrough life you deserve.

Clean Eats   **Buff Body Exercise Plan**

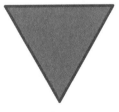

Motivational Mojo

What happens on the inside – your emotions, self-talk, patterns and behaviors – have a direct impact on how you look and feel on the outside. That is why we emphasize so strongly the importance of your inner motivation, or your "mojo," that inner magic that moves us beyond what we thought we could ever do.

Transformation is an inside job. Sure, your *will* and *desire* to succeed are important parts. ***But truly the most important element of the Living Sexy Fit program is fully accepting that you are worthy to live your life all out – and to let your hotness shine like the blazing sun on the Fourth of July.***

"You deserve to melt popsicles, Baby!"

 Let's Start Living Sexy Fit Here!

Let's start by going over the **Five Components** that make up the LSF Lifestyle so you can get going immediately to unleash your Inner Hottie with a <u>Pow</u>! We will go deeper into these subjects throughout the book, and we will revisit topics throughout so you can fully immerse yourself in the Hottie System. I want you to be ragingly successful, so let's go:

1. FACE THE TRUTH – Get Real: Face what is! In the Motivational Mojo chapters, we explore areas in our lives where we frankly have been blowing smoke up our own hineys because we have been too afraid to face the truth. It's time to face the music and accept what IS.

   If you are overweight, out of shape, full of self-loathing and self-doubt, it's now time to be real with yourself and face the piper, because he's not going anywhere until we muster the courage to stop kidding ourselves and blaming others. I know. It's hard. I've been there. But this time you are ready. Can you feel it?

2. RELEASE YOUR BAGGAGE AND LIVE YOUR INNER HOTNESS – It's time to let go, release what no longer serves your Inner Hottie, and step out of the way of your "crazy-spicy" that is ready to be reborn.

OK, so you faced the music and now you have to figure out what luggage, emotionally speaking, you are carrying that you have to give the old heave-ho. People, habits, behaviors, and things. It's amazing how much energy we spend on relationships, emotions, and things well past their expiration dates. Decide if it is worth it to re-up the contract or is it time to switch carriers altogether? Face the fact that it is now time for the loving and gentle boot. You are worthy of great things; dimming your light for anyone or anything is no longer an option.

3. CELEBRATION – Celebrate and Radiate: Your Runway Awaits! A big part of the Living Sexy Fit Lifestyle is "getting it," that we are here to celebrate the uniqueness of who we are. These bodies we were given, even with their imperfections and battle wounds, are still to be celebrated.

   And if we cannot celebrate us, who will?

   Now is your time to shine and live your amazing breakthrough life. And <u>THAT</u> is cause for celebration. Confidence is SEXY. To be confident, you have to believe that you can attain your goals and – the best part – KNOW YOU ARE WORTHY OF ATTAINING THEM! Yes, yes!

4. CLEAN EATING – Eat Clean: Self-respect begins at the lips, not the hips! It's time to fuel your machine with clean eats. Eating healthy is a commitment to your highest and best self. You are worth this high level of self-care. You will feel better. Look better. Bring it on!

   Eating well fuels the mind, body and soul. Nutrition is 70% of the LSF game. Embracing this principle will give you the body you want and deserve. You'll throw out the junk and fill your trunk with whole foods that nurture that inner goddess. Smoking, Baby!

5. EXERCISE – Move It: Find your Inner Hottie in your pleasure of motion! How does it happen? We get lulled into thinking that the couch and the clicker are way more important than moving our bodies freely and celebrating our freedom of motion.

   It's time. If you don't use it, you'll lose it. Reconnecting to our joy in moving our bodies in ways that reflect our inner beauty is a gift that we squander. This is no longer an option for you. Through a combination of weight training and cardiovascular exercise, we will crank the furnaces of our Hottie love machines!

Life is a Journey! We don't call the PRESENT the PRESENT for nothing! Unwrap your gifts and DO YOUR DAY, THIS DAY, like nobody's business!

BUT WAIT! STOP! HOLD IT!
I HAVE HEARD IT ALL BEFORE!

"But, Kate, you have no idea how busy I am, how overworked, depressed, exhausted, broke, tired, sore I am!"

My answer is, "Oh, yes, I do!"

As a single mom of three, a bikini fitness competitor, and a multimillion-dollar business owner, I totally get that life's challenges – and being perpetually overwhelmed and exhausted – can literally knock us to our knees. Trust me, I get it! This stuff is REAL, and it can weigh us down not only physically, but also emotionally and spiritually.

KATE GETS REAL ON HER OWN BREAKDOWN!

When I think back to that time in my life when I finally cried uncle to a life that felt completely out of control, walking into Hard Nocks Gym and meeting my future trainer Rick, I remember the feelings like it was yesterday.

My self-doubt and self-loathing had reached critical mass – my body no longer felt that it was mine, and my spirit was crushed. What had happened to the old energetic, vivacious me, I wondered? I felt like a shell of myself, so filled with sadness and shame.

I had spent my thirties happily giving birth and caring for my babies – my number one priority was to nurture these cuties. But in the process of full-on mothering, I became unrecognizable, even to myself! I remember looking in the mirror one fateful day and shaking my head and wondering where did she go, that free spirit that I remembered. Even more shocking was the look in my eyes of utter defeat and desperation. How could this have happened?

At that point, I was so disturbed that taking immediate action became completely and absolutely non-negotiable.

Can you relate to this story?

Are you experiencing something similar as you look at yourself in the mirror? Are you experiencing this CRAZY incongruity of knowing that the person who is looking back at you, with the bulges and bags, is in NO WAY a true reflection of who you really are?

Are you hungry enough, disturbed enough, by that image to do what you have to do to release fear and self-loathing and all-out EMBRACE the Inner Hottie who is ready to break out in dance and song?

KATE'S BREAKDOWN TO BREAKTHROUGH!

What I realized at my moment of crisis was that staying in this state was 100% no longer acceptable. I was so **disturbed** by how I felt and what I saw that I took IMMEDIATE and RADICAL action to get my fit and sexy self back, PRONTO!

The five steps I took were as follows:

1. I made a commitment to myself to get back in shape. I wanted to be in the best shape of my life at age 40, so I went all out to do just that. NO MATTER WHAT.
2. I joined a gym, not a health spa. Hard Nocks had old equipment and the same Godsmack CD on continual replay. The place was filled with die-hard gym types, often smelly and grunting loudly. I was convinced that my first crush, Rocky, would be stepping through the door at any moment and, hey, I wanted to be ready! Ha!
3. I hired a trainer who saw the "fire" in my eyes and kept me on task. He scared me, and I needed to be scared – trust me! He saw something in me that I didn't. I wanted to understand what that was.
4. I shifted my diet in a big way. More protein, fewer carbs. Food became a fuel and less of a way to soothe myself emotionally.
5. I got my family and friends on board who were ready to support me. Either they're with you as you begin your transformation or they're not. It became really clear, painfully clear, who were my supporters and who were my saboteurs. Was this part easy? Nope. Was it necessary? Hell yeah!

If I can do this, so can you!

Results: HUGE!
Challenging: HELL YEAH!
Satisfaction: DELICIOUS!
Goal achieved: YOU BE THE JUDGE!

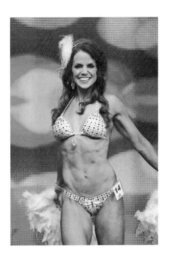

KATE'S BIG TRUTH:

The reason I tell my story is because, behind all the glitz and glamour of the bikini photo above, is a woman (ME!) who fought like H-E Double Hockey Sticks to earn my place on that stage, despite my brother's tragic murder, my gut-wrenching divorce, and my own soul-sucking personal transformation of a woman enmeshed in so much self-doubt and self-loathing I could have sunk the Titanic. Truth!

So this is why, my Living Sexy Fit Goddesses, I am 100% committed to being a part of your success. Because I understand the journey, and there is nothing I am more excited about than your amazing, awe-inspiring, and head-turning transformation.

Whoot, whoot!!! Here we go...

KATE'S DAILY HABIT TIP:
I eat pretty much the same thing every day for breakfast.
I eat 2 whole eggs and a total of 4 egg whites and ½ cup cooked oats with ¼ cup of blueberries for breakfast. Yummo!

Living Sexy Fit   by Kate McKay

PART TWO

Living Sexy Fit

Motivational Mojo

Living Sexy Fit   by Kate McKay

CHAPTER 4

Motivational Mojo – *From the Inside Out*

GETTING TO YOUR "WHY" SO YOU CAN LIVE YOUR BRILLIANCE!
FIGURING OUT WHAT TURNS YOU ON!

Usually the first response I get when I tell people I am 50 years old is, "No way!" Then they often ask my advice about a new diet pill or other shortcuts they can take to get skinny or get ripped. They want to believe so desperately that there must a newfangled diet or certain exercise machine out there that will get them sexy and buff lickety-split.

"Well, isn't there?? I read about it in *People* magazine..." "Saw it on *Dr. Oz*..." "My friend just told me about it..."

When people find out that the key to my success has been simple clean eating and exercise, they are clearly disappointed. I can almost hear their inner dialogue saying dejectedly, "That will never be me; I could never do that."

Screech!!! And I implore, "Why not?"

Why not YOU? Why not?

Why is it that so many of us resign ourselves to mediocre lifestyles? Why do we settle for status quo or good enough?? And on the flipside of this question is the real juice: What does it take to motivate and inspire people who do succeed in getting their sexy back?

What I have found true for my clients who have been successful in attaining their fitness and lifestyle goals—what motivated them to take the plunge and make the changes necessary to live a kick-ass life—is what they describe as an <u>internal</u> shift that expanded their sense of possibility in themselves.

This is cool stuff and worth expanding on with greater detail.

Listen up…

Internal vs. External Motivators

What's the Diff??

Wouldn't it be great if we could "just do it," as Nike proclaims? Unfortunately, understanding what motivates people to get fit and lose weight often precludes the "just do it" mentality.

People are motivated by all kinds of things: looking more attractive, fitting into a wedding dress, impressing peers, proving to the family that they have the will power to succeed, and so on.

And what do all these things have in common? These are all extrinsic, or external, motivators that are concerned with how other people perceive us.

And guess what? These external motivators are much less likely to stick. Because it's not enough to make the shift for someone else – we need to want it for ourselves.

External/Extrinsic Motivators
20% of the motivational game
Engaging in an activity to alter behavior in order to earn an external reward or praise (or to avoid punishment!)

Intrinsic, or internal, motivators are driven by our desire to live more in line with our own values, the essential nature of who we are. I continually ask my clients about their own personal visions – what is it that drives them on a daily basis? Everyone has a unique plan; my job as a fitness coach is to help foster and encourage my clients' dreams. I then get the pleasure of watching them unfold.

Internal/Intrinsic Motivators
80% of the motivational game
Taking pleasure in an activity driven by an inner sense of reward or accomplishment

---

What about you? What is it that you want for yourself? How will your life be different when you're living your life more in line with your own values? How will you feel when you achieve your fitness and weight-loss goals? Who are you with? What are you doing? What season is it? What are you wearing? The more you can fill in the blanks, the clearer the vision and the closer you will be to living the life you deserve.

Getting to the truth of your "why" in your motivational mojo is the secret to success not only in your fitness goals but in all areas of your life.

There is no magic bullet (yet) to getting fit and losing weight. However, spending a few moments to think of what will internally motivate you to embrace positive change is worth its weight in gold.

Sometimes you just have to let go and give yourself permission to live your dream and be your best. But why is this so hard to do?

GET REAL: FACING WHAT IS!

As I shared with you in the last chapter, I completely get how our inner self-perception wreaks havoc on our sizzle. I have been there and done that, but I am here to tell you it doesn't have to be that way. So let's dig deeper into the process and get busy with the tools on how to get REAL, get RADICAL, and unleash YOUR LIVING SEXY FIT SELF that is so ready to GO, GO, GO!

Resistance to facing the music of our past is often what really causes diets to fail and exercise plans to get left by the wayside. Our commitment falls away when the negative self-talk rears its ugly head.

Made to feel "less than" and ashamed when you were 5?
 Your body remembers.
Called fat when you were 12?
 That memory is still lodged.
Crushed in a love relationship?
 Yup, your body got that stored as well.

KATE NEWS FLASH:

Our bodies store old memories, like bulletproof vaults, whether we remember these experiences consciously or not, emotional wounds affix to our bodies like Velcro.

As a coach, I see this physically manifested all the time in my clients: upper-back pain, hip tightness, and shoulder tears. Often our injuries have emotional components that we have stuffed away in our memory banks.

And how do we cope? We use alcohol, food, sex, and other addictive habits and behaviors to stuff them down and away so we don't have to deal with them.

As Dr. Phil asks so succinctly, "How is that working for you?"

It's not!

That's why you are ready to take action! To release, to let go, so that you can embrace that inner sexy swagger and live the life you WANT and, more important, DESERVE!

I'm personally committed, from the bottom of my soul, to ensuring that it happens for you so let's get busy!

But before we move on, remember: Any nasty thing that was spoken to you or the yucky way people made you feel was their issue, NOT YOURS!

The quicker you get this, the faster your Inner Hottie will pop and come back alive!

You are worth it! I know you're committed. So let's jump in and make a commitment today and stay on fire all the way to the end.

1. What do you really want? I mean really want, with a burning in your belly that you may even be embarrassed to say out loud? Time to say it out loud and put it down on paper. Say bye-bye to playing small!

2. What are you committed to? There's a big difference between just being interested in something and being completely committed. I don't do "just interested," for the record. Do you want a good life or a great one? Do you want to be cool or smoking hot? Thought so. Write down what you're committed to on your hotness journey.

3. OK, so why are you committed to your fitness? "What??" Yup, I mean WHY? You have to know the WHY because from the WHY comes the motivation and the action. Remember this is YOUR "WHY," not someone else's! Go ahead and write! Don't skip over this!

4. Are you ready to take immediate action to take your Sexy Fit Self off the back burner of your life?

5. Why? Yup, that question again! Write your answers down! Why are you ready to take your Sexy Fit Self off the back burner?

Excellent job! This work is not easy but is so important in attaining the freedom that the Living Sexy Fit Lifestyle provides.

Now, let's move onto some fun stuff: celebrating your inner confidence and showing the world what you got going on!

(Wow! Look at you with all that mojo!!)

Staying Positive in a Largely Negative World!

Exude Confidence for the Sexy Glow!!

The key ingredient to success in my life, and I guarantee it will be in yours, is this: "Attitude is everything." You see, by focusing on the positive, we can do all the right exercises we need and eat all the right foods. But if we're stressed out or angry in our approach to life, we'll never—and I mean never—get the results we desire.

You see, nothing—and I mean nothing—opens the channels of healing and vitality more than gratitude and positive attitude. If you want amazing results from your training program, bring amazing energy. How will you act, stand, breathe, and move when you are living in a body with the spirit that you desire? What will you be doing, who will you be with, and how will you feel when you are celebrating that ultimate success?

Exude confidence. Just being confident draws people in and *to* you. A more *confident* you is a more *charismatic* you. And sometimes in the beginning, you just have to fake it until you make it, especially if you are trying something for the first time.

You are a unique person with unique gifts and talents. The best thing to do is to be YOU, not some cheap imitation of you. Is Julia Roberts the most beautiful woman in the world? The best actress? How about Sandra Bullock, Tony Robbins, or Ellen DeGeneres? What makes them so attractive is their inner confidence and hottie mojo that draws us in. They are hot, and they know they are hot, despite their imperfections! How cool is that?

What we may perceive as our weaknesses and try to hide only get in the way of our shining full on, especially when it is time to hit the stage or move into a new experience. Did I have what it took to build a multimillion-dollar business without taking a single business class in my life? By all appearances, um, hell no! But you better believe I walked and talked like I did until I was living it! You can, too.

You are human! Don't be afraid of your humanness! People want to see the real you, not some phony imitation!

Celebrate Your Best YOU by Bringing Your Uniqueness to the World!

It is not always easy to define yourself, and that's why I think it is so important to work with a coach you trust to help you bring out YOU with a "Pow!" A coach or mentor will help you draw out what makes you unique and, as a result, bring greater success in all aspects in your life.

Sometimes that means being clear on where your strengths lie. But often it is much more subtle, like understanding that you need to get out of your own way so your authenticity and uniqueness can shine.

So many of us understand that we shouldn't dim others' lights by living in judgment of who they are, but we usually don't give ourselves the same courtesy.

It is my belief that we are all here for a divine assignment, something that is uniquely "you." My question is, who are you to play small and dim your own light? Well, who are you??

This is not necessarily the easiest process, but it is a crucial step in bringing the charismatic and sexy YOU front and center. Be kind to yourself in the process, and embrace the imperfect and evolving you. There is no dress rehearsal. Live all out each and every day like this is your final rodeo. You can never get this beautiful moment back.

This is the energy I want you to take forth throughout your day. Share your enthusiasm with others. It's contagious.

And remember, when you bump into people who have bad attitudes, that shouldn't affect you at all. Understand that it's them and not you. Stay in your greatness. Be sure to share your hopes and dreams with those who will support you on your journey. Most important, enjoy the ride!

Celebrate your positivity.
Remember, attitude is everything. And confidence is sexy!

Tidbit: Daily micro-steps lead to your kick-ass life. Achieving your fitness and health goals is just adding DAILY ACTION to your dreams. You can do this!

 Hottie Hazard – Not Getting Enough Shut-Eye!

Confession: This is the hardest hazard for me to avoid, and I am sure this is true for many of you. Life is so full and busy – and, darn it, we don't want to miss a thing!

But the bottom line is this: Your Living Sexy Fit factor needs replenishing daily, and that means putting your beautiful temple to rest! The latest studies show that the lean people out there sleep more than the less lean. Sleep-deprived peeps just have less control over their food choices

– that's a fact. I know that when I'm tired, the first thing I want is sugar, and lots of it! Can you relate?

Another factoid: Getting less sleep decreases our bodies' ability to regulate glucose levels, which in turn increases insulin production, leading to weight gain and a boatload of other scary health issues.

EEK! Please don't let that be you!

So, sleep, rest, restore. You deserve it, and your inner Living Sexy Fit self will thank you with more joy, increased energy and a stronger and fitter body to fuel you throughout the day.

Making your health and hotness a priority takes passion and commitment. Avoiding living-fit hazards will get you where you want to go quicker and with greater energy and vitality than you can imagine.

Keep moving. Stay in action. Eat clean and make your life amazing!

CHAPTER 5

Motivational Mojo: Tolerations – *Giving a Boot to Your Hot Mess!*

ARE YOU READY TO HAVE MASSIVE FREEDOM AND TO LET YOUR INNER HOTTIE SHINE ALL OUT?

By zapping tolerations, you will gain freedom and fun. And <u>THAT</u> is the sizzling-hot truth!

TOLERATIONS: little or sometimes big things that you have been tolerating in your life that eat away little pieces of your confidence, pleasure, happiness, and joy.

And guess who is responsible for all that?

Yup, YOU!

I'd say it is due time you let some of these pesky buggers go, wouldn't you agree?

By zapping tolerations, you will immediately experience the following:

- less stress
- increased productivity
- easier relationships
- healthier boundaries
- increased self-esteem and self-worth
- inner glow and greater flow

So, what is standing in your way of living a full-on juicy life? Be honest with yourself. What changes are you ready to take because you are now ready to roll?

Below, please list at least 10 changes you're willing to make. Continue on as long as you like so you can put them all out there. This is like having your own bitch session – from this point, you are going to be your own bestie. Start zapping these stressors so you can start living your life with greater sizzle and increased energy to boot.

This really works! Trust me!

Some examples of tolerations: no help with housework, a disorganized desk, lack of sleep, disrespectful children, a poor relationship with your partner, being overweight and out of shape, cluttered drawers, a dirty car, negative self-talk, credit card debt, holey underwear. You name it. Now it's time for you to let it rip!

1.
2.
3.

4.

5.

6.

7.

8.

9.

10.

Great! Now review your list and circle the top three that you are ready to take action on. Write them down here:

1.

2.

3.

Excellent job. Now it is time to create a strategy to rid yourself of these tolerations that are sucking you dry.

What are you prepared to do today to deal with these tolerations and live a less stressful and more joy-filled life? Write your ideas below. Please don't skip this part! Go!

1.

2.

3.

Congratulations! You have committed to TAKE ACTION to Live Sexy Fit all out! I am so proud of you!

Celebrate and Radiate!

KATE NEWS FLASH: The process of moving into your GREATNESS is wonderful, amazing, and a little scary, too! Be prepared for all of it!

What I realized was that as I up-leveled my life and moved into my "BIG," the part that scared me the most was not knowing who I was going to be if I wasn't my self-loathing and self-doubting self! Who knew that was the BIGGEST FEAR I had that was keeping my fit self on the back burner of life???

You are the life of your own party, and it is due time you start to **Live It**!

AND THE RESULT: Be prepared to have people drawn to you who normally wouldn't even have said hello to you before. Cute members of the opposite sex, dogs, old people at the grocery store. THIS JUST HAPPENS!

You see, when you are at peace and loving on yourself for who you are, and just doing your THANG without being concerned about what others think or being crushed by your own self-judgment, YOU SHINE, plain and simple.

This is not about EGO.

This is not about being phony.

This is about being fully YOU, the powerful YOU, the silly YOU, the vulnerable YOU. YOU.

This is about living in your true and authentic self, because when we celebrate ourselves, our uniqueness, our beauty in and out, the world shifts, PEOPLE!

I promise you this! You'll find smiles, laughter, prosperity, abundance, kisses, parking spots, YOU NAME IT!

Also, and so important: By celebrating your Living Sexy Fit self, you serve as a positive role model to others: your kids, friends, intimate partners. This is what authenticity and integrity look like, and I am telling you that it is AMAZING!

Go be your SEXY FIT SELF, and carry your inner celebration with you wherever you go.

With a sparkle in my eye, and knowing that you are so completely and totally worth it, I celebrate YOU!

"The opposite of courage is not fear but inaction.
Stay in action! Success happens one micro-step at a time!"

The power of Living Sexy Fit is embracing your inner confidence so you can shine at your highest wattage. You are here on this planet to be a bright light. Stop dimming your glow!

Keep a record of your inner reflections and changes in a journal, and also record and celebrate compliments and encouragement you receive from others. They'll serve as reminders when you experience those not-so-sexy days when you are feeling more icy cold than spicy hot. Such days could be happier, but you will live through them as long as you keep leaning in and moving into your beautiful Inner Hottie, who cannot wait to be released.

Living Sexy Fit | by Kate McKay

Motivational Mojo – *Revisiting the Holistic Approach to Your Health and Hotness!*

Being so active in the public eye as a fitness coach, trainer, and athlete, I'm often approached by people who want to ask about losing weight. They often think that, hey, all I need to do is lose weight and my whole entire life will just be rocking all the way around. EEK! Not necessarily!!!

That's like saying that people who win the lottery are happier than the rest of us because now they don't have money worries. Nonsense! How could you explain, then, the number of winners who end up bankrupt and divorced after they burn through their entire bankroll?

This is the honest truth.

Money doesn't buy happiness, and neither does skinny.

The fact is that people who end up rocking their weight loss really do experience a full life transformation that changes their entire way of perceiving themselves and their relationships.

You see, it isn't just about the weight! It's a LIFESTYLE.

What these successful dieters have found is that the transformation they were seeking occurred from the inside out. They were ready to release self-defeating patterns and behaviors that kept them in bodies that really did not reflect who they were on the inside.

Living Sexy Fit is an inside job. To experience rock-star-quality transformation, we have to change how we experience our own realities before we hit the rocking runways of life.

So, how about you? What changes have you decided to take on to let go of and embrace the new you?

We know who we are, deep, deep in our souls, if we really listen. When what's reflected on the outside doesn't match what's on the inside, we're filled with unrest and unease. We overeat, stress out, toss and turn at night, and bitch and complain because we know we are not living in our best and highest selves. We just know it!

The Living Sexy Fit Lifestyle is about bringing into balance our inner and outer mojos so we can live lives of integrity – body, mind, and soul. This is good stuff! You can do this.

The fact is that you are worthy of having your body reflect that inner you, that strong, sexy, and vibrant spirit that lies within, waiting to be reborn. You're worthy of it – and the world's ready to see YOU. Today is the day to take on the challenge of living your greatest and best life yet!

 Hottie Hazard – Skipping Meals. Hey, I'm Not Hungry!

Nothing, and I mean nothing, makes me feel LESS HOT than when I crash mid-day from lack of proper nutrition. YUCK!

You know what I am talking about: that 3 p.m. crash when you feel like you have fallen and can't get back up, and reach for a Snickers and a Coke because that has been your past cure-all to lift you up (and eventually throw up, due a poor eating cycle).

The real deal? Starving yourself typically backfires. When you don't fuel your machine, your body goes into starvation mode and your metabolism slows to a trickle.

Then what happens next? You binge at night on calorie-laden food. And guess what? Your body stores those extra yum-yum calories as FAT!

To attain and maintain a lean and sexy body, start with breakfast every day. I don't care if you are not hungry or don't like breakfast – yakety-yack. Just do it! Please! Your body will thank you.

Living Sexy Fit   by Kate McKay

CHAPTER 7

Motivational Mojo – *Why Living a Life of Integrity Is Sexy*

Integrity: adherence to moral principles; honesty; wholeness.

To be our best, we must be whole. That is, we have to be responsible for our actions and inactions, respond honestly and fully in our conversations, honor our bodies and ourselves, and respect our relationships and our environments.

When you are **in a state of Integrity**, you experience these:
- less conflict
- more self-acceptance
- consistent feeling of peace, health, and emotional balance
- nonreactive state of being

When you are **out of Integrity**, you experience these:
- continual disturbances
- frustrations

- conflict in relationships
- self-sabotage
- distress

"Do not build obstacles in your imagination." —Norman Vincent Peale

Well, darn it, how in the heck can we be in integrity in our lives when 70% of our thoughts are unconscious?

The answer? We have to work super, super hard to counteract the negative talk that sabotages our efforts to be fit and lose weight by paying close attention to our thoughts and feelings and to how we show up in our relationships to others.

The challenge is that, when we get all excited about a great opportunity or about an awesome dream and vision for ourselves and our future, our own unconscious minds go overboard and start bashing away at joy and excitement.

Yup, we are the ones who cause the greatest damage to our hopes and dreams.

Not your mom, your dad, your boss, your spouse, your kids. YOU!

"Choose today to no longer sit on the sidelines of your own life."

So many of us go so far in life and then we put our car in park! Are you parked? Are your hopes and dreams stopped in a traffic jam that you yourself created? Are you frozen in fear and have the foot pressed on the brake instead of the accelerator of your life?

Are you in a dead-end job? Do you accept a fat and out-of-shape body as your norm? Are you living in a lifeless, passionless relationship? Feeling spiritually empty? Isn't it time to put your car into gear and drive?

No one ever became great by imitation. Imitation is limitation.
Dare to be who you are!

What are you giving up to play it safe and live small? Living a life outside of integrity keeps fear alive. Fear is just a condition that your mind makes up to keep you parked. You have to decide that you are no longer interested in playing small, in living a life *less than*. There is only one life designed just for you. YOURS! Dare to live the best version of you!

Please answer the questions about integrity below. Please don't skip this part!!

1. What does the word integrity mean to you?

2. How do you know when you are in integrity?

3. When you are not in integrity – how do you know?

4. What does your body tell you/how do you feel?

5. What does your mind tell you/what are the stories or dialogues that replay?

Again, knowledge is power! The more you know, the better you grow.

Your path to greatness will not always be clear. But don't let your vision be clouded in fear and doubt. You are here for great things. Don't settle for small. Live BIG or go home.
If you find an excuse, choose not to pick it up!

Don't spend your creative energy thinking up lame excuses why you CANNOT do what you know you MUST do.

Say "HELL NO!" to stinkin' thinkin'!

Stinkin' Thinkin': old ways of thinking about who you are that keep you stuck and playing small!

Time to hit the delete button on your old stories that no longer serve you!

Stay in action. Eat clean, exercise, and keep pressing through fear by filling your thoughts with positive affirmation and your clear-cut action plan for success. Be crystal clear on what you ultimately want.

Dream BIG, and EXPECT AMAZING OUTCOMES! Also, you can expect detours, roadblocks, and hazards in the road. Not one of them will be something you cannot overcome. Not one!

If you believe with this conviction, you will move mountains. Believe this!

Choose to be open to possibility. Choose to say yes!

 Hottie Hazard – Jumping on the Latest Fad Diet Bandwagon

Sorry, but there is no magic pill or restricted food diet (lemon water and egg whites, anyone?) that will quickly melt away your extra weight and keep it off.

Lifestyle switch-up is the only sure-shot way to create long-lasting change. Stay with the basics of eating clean 80% to 90% of the time, eat smaller portions with greater frequency, and get that bootie moving every day! This is the magic combo.

CHAPTER 8

Motivational Mojo: Getting Clear – *Creating Healthy Relationships with Yourself and Others*

WHAT THE HECK IS HAPPENING?
UNDERSTANDING YOUR EMOTIONS THROUGH YOUR TRANSFORMATION

As you move through your Living Sexy Fit transformation, you will experience some emotions that are best addressed at the outset:

1. unexplained emotional fogginess
2. clarity of ideas that shock you
3. intolerance of people lying and not being straight-shooters
4. hurt feelings that seem out of context with the given situation
5. moments of bliss that you just can't explain
6. uncontrollable laughter

7. uncontrollable tears
8. peace
9. joy
10. relief

You just start feeling different.

Really different.

And you can't quite put your finger on what it is!

People around you notice it, too, and are not quite sure what has happened either. Where is the "old" you?

Congratulations! You are moving into a transformational period where your old ways of being no longer serve you, and your greater calling—the Bigger and Better YOU—is waiting to be born! Welcome!

This is the moment you have been waiting for. So why does it feel so... strange?

As your coach, I am here to help you, support you, and challenge you through this crazy stage as you set out to live your breakthrough life. You are going to be fine. More than fine – you are going to be amazing.

Let's go over some strategies you can use to make this easier for you and those who surround you, and we will start with talking some more about these emotions in transformation.

First, even though certain reactions you experience may seem out of context, know that sometimes—if a particular issue is laden with emotional wounds that have not been addressed, holding a whole history of emotional hurts—you may unknowingly react completely out of context to the actual event at hand.

For example:

Your spouse is late, without calling, and shows up just after you have put dinner on the table. You flip out.

or:

Your business partner sent out a proposal that you had not yet reviewed and given your stamp of approval. You seethe.

Reactions? Normal. Why is that, you may ask??

What is happening is that old wounds are surfacing so you can resolve them once and for all. If tardiness or not getting a say in something that is important to you really truly matters, then you are being faced with a great opportunity to clear that up head-on, so you can live in a new level of integrity and clarity.

Make sense?

This is called <u>creating healthy boundaries</u> and maintaining a higher level of self-care. This is about being clear on what is acceptable to you, without judgment of others, so you are more aligned truly with your authentic self. Bravo!

Will there be bumps on the way? Sure.

Will you perhaps need to say you're sorry a few times? Perhaps.

Will others be clear on what is important to you and why? Absolutely.

Congratulations for putting your integrity of self at the center of your Living Sexy Fit transformation. It takes some work, but the steps you take here and now are not only invaluable, they are essential to your transformation.

Again, understand that transformation, adapting new ways of being and communicating, stirs up some real juicy stuff. It surfaces now with such power and intensity because this is a reminder of what you must release to be finally free of your past. And this, my friend, is way good.

To be clear: When you are in the midst of it, it may not feel good. But soon the clarity and release you experience will be so worth it. I promise. I have worked with many people who have been challenged through this scenario. You will make it through, as well, more powerful and focused than ever.

As you move into a higher level of integrity, your goals become more attainable. You feel an overall greater sense of peace, and you experience an increased sense of abundance. Your relationships are richer. Success occurs with less effort and more ease.

Now, doesn't that sound like it will so be worth it??

Important Self Care Tip: Talk issues out with your coach, therapist, or accountability partner. Write in a journal or meditate, but do not give up on your Living Sexy Fit dream and fail to face the work that your breakthrough life requires.

Often, quitters are more concerned with how far they have to go versus how far they have come. That is not YOU. You are not a quitter!

Stay clear on your goals, choose action over reaction, and stay in self-love and self-acceptance. Picture how you want conversations to end up and hold steady on that vision. Be less worried about being right. Be most concerned with staying in your integrity and in grace.

Congratulations for digging in and committing to your highest and best vision of you!

Please review the eliciting questions below. Who are you now, as you read through and answer these questions? Some answers may surprise you. Be kind in your reactions, as emotions can come up that have been latent for maybe years…

As you think about your transformation, ask the following:

1. What are some things that could get in the way of achieving your goals and living a breakthrough Living Sexy Fit life?

2. Are there people you think may not support your personal Living Sexy Fit transformation?

3. Why?

4. Please list 3 people who you believe will support your Living Sexy Fit dream.

5. Ask yourself this: if you do not attain your goals and dreams, what do you lose? Are you willing to take that risk?

Tidbits from Kate:

Want to increase your Happiness Quotient?

Give a little sugar to the three tidbits below:

1. Appreciation: digging what you have, seeing what it is. Just like a big hug, appreciation asks for nothing and gives everything. Try it.

2. Personal Power: taking responsibility for what is yours and taking action on living a JUICY life. Responsibility by action. Wow. Look out, cookout.

3. Leading with Your Strength: What makes your heart skip when you do it? What did you love when you were 5 years old? What do people keep telling you you're really good at? Okay, now go ahead and do more of it. Building up your weaknesses while diminishing your strengths is so old school.

Want to really boost your personal strength knowledge times 10? Buy the book *Strengths Finder 2.0*, take the test at the end of the book, and be awed by the many ways you rock. This test changed my life, really! Check it out.

**Celebrate each and every small change/success
in your body that you can see, feel and relish.**

The heart of motivation – your inner sexy fit fuel – is your internal body-soul feedback, which is what fuels what I call Living Sexy Fit mojo. Living in celebration from the inside out.

Again, is it going to be easy? Hell no! Is it going to be worth it? Hell yes!!

Keep a record of your inner reflections and changes in a journal, and also record and celebrate compliments and encouragement you receive from others. They'll serve as reminders when you experience those not-so-sexy days when you are feeling more icy cold than spicy hot. Such days could be happier, but you will live through them as long as you keep leaning in and moving into your beautiful Inner Hottie, who cannot wait to be released.

CHAPTER 9

Motivational Mojo – *Action Plan to Living Sexy Fit*

LIVING YOUR UNIQUE VISION AND CREATING A LIFE OF YOUR DREAMS

We were all put on this beautiful planet, in this abundant world, for a REASON, each of us unique. We all desire to be self-defined. So why do we spend so much time letting others define it for us?

The best part of unleashing your Inner Hottie is finally understanding that this whole process is an inside job: to discover your life purpose, to live in abundance, to revel in self-love and acceptance, and to serve at your highest level in your greatest good!

You cannot live this way if you are letting someone else write the agenda. You are in charge of writing your own script! What stories do you want to be telling someday from your rocking chair? Come on! Make them juicy, exciting, and HOT!!

To unleash your Inner Sexy Fit requires DAILY ACTION STEPS so you can hit your Hottie bulls-eye. Sure, crappy things happen. Even tragedy will strike your life and knock you to your knees. But if you develop your resilience muscle and keep self-love and acceptance at the core of how you live on a daily basis, you will be AMAZED by how your life looks and feels.

I want is that for you: Joy and peace and a burning SIZZLE that keep your life roaring with passion and desire because you are living in DAILY ACTION to live your best and most JUICY LIFE!

Now, a juicy life requires you to take decisive action, so let's get you busy...

Why is creating a life vision so important?

Because creating a vision statement is the framework necessary to creating a powerful and amazing life! It provides the direction necessary to how you live each and every day.

Picture this:

Goals, Wants, Needs →

Mission, Purpose →

Vision! →

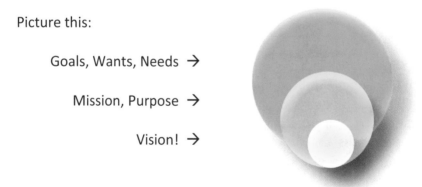

At the center of you is your vision, your Inner Hottie target bulls-eye. That is what your ideal life is going to look like when you are living your life all in. This is where the good stuff starts and ends.

Let's start with creating your Living Sexy Fit vision!

Screeech! Loud braking sound!

**"Help! I'm Ready to Make a Big Change,
but I Don't Know How to Start!"**

So you are ready to make a big change in how you live your life, but you just cannot figure out where to start.

I hear it all the time.

What happens is, because we don't put a plan and structure around our dream, our commitment wavers. And then the stinkin' thinkin' cycle begins anew, and BAM, we find our head in the fridge looking to feed our disappointment and disgust.

Why do we keep doing this?

Well, unless you have a crystal clear vision of what you want and how your life will be different when you achieve it, you will end up beating yourself to a pulp because all you see and experience is your failure.

So can we all agree to stop this nonsense?

Kate's Behavior Modification Tip: Sometimes we just have to go Pavlov and create a physical action that breaks up our negative thinking. I go right to breathing. I breathe in peace and blow out anxiety. Trust me, you can regain PEACE in one breath! Pick an action that works for you, such as tapping on your thigh, rubbing between your eyes, pushing into your palm. Create an action that centers you. Make this a habit to restore your inner peace.

"So, Kate, what is a Vision Statement, anyway??"

Vision Statement: A guiding light that shines in the darkness, illuminating your hopes and dreams. Your vision statement is a written description of how you want to live your most amazing life. It serves as a *guideline* for how you live every day.

To create a vision that motivates, encourages and drives you, consider the following:

1. What is the most positive and affirming mental image you can create of yourself in the not-too-far-off future?

2. Where are you?

3. What are you doing?

4. Who are you with?

5. What are you wearing?

6. How is the weather?

7. What emotions are you experiencing as you celebrate your Living Sexy Fit life?

Ready, Set, GO!

OK, now it is time to put pen to paper and write down IN DETAIL your vision for yourself, including what you will be doing and who you will be with, what the weather is like, how you are feeling, when you are living the Sexy Fit Lifestyle:

.

- Be sure to write in present tense, as though you have accomplished your vision.
- Write about things you enjoy doing on a daily basis.
- Write about what you value.
- Write about what fulfills you.

In my amazing Living Sexy Fit vision, I am

LIVE THIS EXPERIENCE IN YOUR BODY, MIND AND SOUL!

Living Sexy Fit Goal Implementation!

"All our dreams can come true, if we have the courage to pursue them."
~ Walt Disney

Now that you have created a vision statement, it is time to add some spark by putting your dream into action. Start by reviewing your vision statement and extracting two to three events that you can create some action steps around to bring your sexy sizzle to center stage.

Remember: A Goal Is Just a Dream with a Timeline!

A goal needs to be realistic and measurable. Now, when I say realistic, I mean that if your goal is to lose weight, don't create some unrealistic goal such as losing 10 pounds for the weekend or running a marathon at the end of the month when you haven't walked farther than your mailbox in years.

I hate to burst your bubble, but a healthy and realistic weight loss goal is roughly 1 to 2 lbs. a week. Planning for more than that will unfortunately be setting yourself up for failure and disappointment. Please don't do that. I want you to succeed, so let's be sure to set up goals that you can nail.

Putting a timeline on your goals is another crucial element to Living Sexy Fit. Working within a timeline will require you to stay in action on a daily basis. Action breeds success! Your daily habits create your reality. If you are ready to up-level your life and live with full-on inner sass, make the commitment to put a period on the date of accomplishment. You deserve it.

Let's create a timeline for your goal:

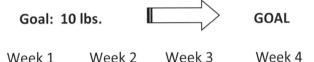

Goal: 10 lbs.   **GOAL**

Week 1   Week 2   Week 3   Week 4

Start with the end in mind, making the goal juicy and exciting.

Sample goals: lose fat, gain muscle, develop six-pack abs. What's yours? Be specific!

Using the Power of Intention to Transform Your Life by Setting B.I.G. Goals!

Resolution vs. Intention

Why do so many people fail at living their New Year's resolutions to get fit and lose weight? The truth is, it is not enough to *resolve* to do something, to will it into existence. We need to add the power of *intention* behind our vision and our goals.

You see, it takes more than just powerful THOUGHTS to have a breakthrough life. We must also have powerful FEELINGS and ACTIONS. That is why we must fully embrace the "WHY" in our commitment to Living Sexy Fit.

When choosing goals to fire into action, consider the following:

1. Choose a JUICY one!
    *   Determine a specific and juicy goal!
    *   Don't skimp on your dream!
    *   This is your life! Make it delicious!

2. Make it **B.I.G**!
   B – Bodacious
   I – Irresistible
   G – Glorious

   If it doesn't excite you, scratch it!

3. Write it down!
   Add all the goods to this goal, fully imagining what it will feel like to be living IN the success of the accomplishment.

4. Share it with someone who can hold you ACCOUNTABLE.
   Select these people carefully! They will become the keepers of your dream and will be instrumental in keeping you to the fire. Especially when you wake up someday and just don't feel like it, or whatever trick your mind decides to play!

5. Break it down!
   Break it down to micro-steps and put some bookmarks on it. Give your goal some sugar!

   - **Example – Goal: To lose 5 lbs. in 28 days**
        Action: I will stick 100% to the Eat Clean Diet 80/20 rule
        Action: I will exercise every day for at least 30 minutes
        Action: I will book a mani/pedi for day 29 to celebrate my achievement
        Milestone: I will have achieved a 3-lb. weight loss by day 16

Now it is your turn. Go ahead! Write it down! Remember: Juicy goals! Not lame ones!

Goal 1
   Action
   Action
   Action
     Milestone

Goal 2
   Action
   Action
   Action
     Milestone

Goal 3
   Action
   Action
   Action
     Milestone

"Success! Have it <u>Your</u> way!"

Hottie Hazard – Oops! Missed My Workout! Oh, Well... Not!

Your Inner Hottie News Flash: Moving that bod of yours is NON-NEGOTIABLE, if you <u>really</u> want it. You said you wanted it, didn't you? I could have sworn I heard you say that you wanted it BAD...

Staying committed to your Living Sexy Fit vision is not going to be easy, but it will be worth it. Anyway, I have never heard of anyone saying, "Shoot, I regret working out today." Not ever.

CHAPTER 10

Motivational Mojo: Fear and Resistance – *Being Your Own Stick in the Mud and How to BREAK THROUGH Using the Power of Affirmation*

"I JUST CAN'T SEEM TO GET OUT OF MY OWN WAY!"
"IT'S HARD FOR ME TO STAY POSITIVE."

Studies show it takes 21 to 28 days to establish a new habit, so expect resistance and challenges at the beginning of putting the Living Sexy Fit Lifestyle into action!

The bigger and bolder your new vision is, the greater the likelihood that you will experience internal resistance and fear. Your unconscious mind does not always play fair. Expect some dirty pool!

This is when having completed your **Vision Statement** comes into play in a big way! Please keep at it and stay on track!

You will soon reach the wonderful place, the tipping point, where you begin to experience the positive benefits of lifestyle change that far outweigh your old and outdated habits that have kept you out of the red-hot zone.

Stay committed even when you want to quit. The feelings of being overwhelmed will pass! You are worthy of a breakthrough life!

When you're thinking of releasing old habits and adopting new ones, picture a rubber band. The further you pull, the greater the resistance. It's time for you to pick up a bigger band!

Harness the Power of Resistance!

Understand that Resistance is just part of the Living Sexy Fit game! Embrace it!

So, here is a rough description of where our emotions take us on the Living Sexy Fit journey:

☺ Days 1 and 2 – Woo hoo, you are ready to go! You are so excited! You can do this!

☹ 3rd day – not as easy, enthusiasm wanes.

☹ 2nd week – hardest time period. Enthusiasm has left the building. Keep at building new habits! Keep Eating Clean! Keep Moving! YOU CAN DO IT! Quitting is not an option!

☺ 3rd and 4th weeks – a little easier; you start seeing results! "Wow, I feel more energetic." Hey, my face looks thinner." "What happened to my sugar craving?? It is gone!"

Fear – False Expectations Appearing Real!

Your "why?" has to be clear to accomplish your goal.

Are you looking for an excuse to give up? Or are your own trembling fears an opportunity to change and make improvements to your life? Choose the latter!

You are a failure only if you fail to get up or blame someone else for pushing you down. You are bigger than your fear!

Believe in your possibility!

Tapping into Power of Affirmation!
Be Confident in Your Success!

Affirmation: a statement or proposition that is declared to be true.

I am shocked at some of the things I hear people using as "affirmations" for themselves to get motivated, such as, "I don't want to look like a fat pig anymore," "I'm sick of feeling like crap." "I make myself sick." Really?? I am not kidding; these are real, live examples of the stories people tell me when I ask them what motivates them to make a positive lifestyle change.

They want these changes for themselves desperately, and think that they are being positive… AGH!

Creating positive affirmations takes practice. However, if you keep using positive language to state your wishes and intentions, you will discover that dreams really do come true!

Practice saying the affirmations below out loud and see which ones resonate with you – or write down some of your own.

Try these on for size!

- I am worthy of a healthy and fit body!
- I am ready to embrace the Living Sexy Fit lifestyle.
- I deserve all the good that shows up in my life.
- I see myself moving with ease and grace.
- I am ready to live my life full out.
- I am here to do great things!
- My body is a temple worthy of extreme self-care.
- I deserve to feel sexy and strong!
- I am powerful beyond measure.
- I am a bright light in the world.
- I celebrate all that is good about me.
- I forgive myself for any wrongs I have done, perceived or imagined.
- I live in complete integrity in all aspects of my life.
- I am peace, love, and joy in the world.

Your top three:
1.
2.
3.

Kate's Tip: I stick Post-it notes all over my house with affirmations when I am having a tough week. Visual reminders are great cues to keep you aligned with your vision and remind yourself why you are worthy of achieving all that you desire.

Steps you can apply today to activate your inner mojo!

- Start where you are, taking one micro-step at a time.
- Keep practicing saying YES to your possibility! As soon as you hear your negative self-talk, hit the PAUSE button on your gremlins and push PLAY to your possibility. Sometimes tapping on one leg as pause and on the other thigh as play helps re-program your thinking and keeps you in the right lane to your big dream.
- Lighten up! Laugh at yourself! Nothing shifts your experience more than laughter and joy!
- Watch a funny movie.
- Hang with people who lighten your spirit.
- Involve yourself in a community/church that lifts you up.
- Practice random acts of service – surprise others.

The most rewarding thing you can do if you feel stagnant about your lot in life is to open a service station! Nothing lifts us up more than when we serve others.

Great work.

Now it is time onto the Clean Eats section of the Living Sexy Fit Program. Let's go!

PART THREE

The Living Sexy Fit Clean Eats Plan

Living Sexy Fit   by Kate McKay

CHAPTER 11

The Living Sexy Fit Clean Eats Mojo Revealed

What if I told you that to Live Sexy Fit, you would potentially eat more than you are used to? That you would no longer suffer from the 3 p.m. afternoon slump? That you would experience increased vitality and energy?

It's true! And I can't wait to share with you the <u>how-to's</u>!

But First: A Tad More on Kate's Back Story

Twelve years ago, after I gave birth to the last of my three children, my desire to finally get back into shape and leave self-flagellation behind reached critical mass. I was ready to get my body back. So, I hired a trainer named Eric. He wanted me to keep a food log as part of our work together. The first time I turned it in, he said "You are not eating enough."

What? How could that be? I thought I was doing so well! Cripes, I even doctored the log to make me look better to try to impress him.

Wrong.

"Wait! I thought I had done so well over the last few days of food tracking!" I exclaimed.

"Nope, said Eric, shaking his head disappointedly. "Not enough and not the right kinds of foods.

Not enough?? Not the right foods? Humpf. I was insulted!

Pregnant pause...

Okay, maybe he had a point there. I looked at my bloated and swollen body in the mirror that night. Apparently, what I had been doing was not working. I realized then and there that if I wanted my sexy back, it was high time for me to get re-educated to the how-to's of eating clean.

Okay, All Right! So, What _IS_ Clean Eats?

CLEAN EATS is eating foods that fuel YOUR BEAUTIFUL, AMAZING machine, that get your motor running optimally for maximum energy and fat-burning capabilities, so you can live the Sexy Fit Lifestyle!

Sound good? Great, then let's dig in...

CHAPTER 12

The Living Sexy Fit Clean Eats Lifestyle

CLEAN EATS AND EMOTIONAL EATING – REBOOT YOUR STINKIN' THINKIN'!

EATING CLEAN: fueling your machine with self-love and healthy eats to maximize your mojo!

Before we dig into nutrition the Living Sexy Fit way, I would like to address the super-important issue of how so many of us use food to soothe instead of fuel our bodies and souls.

The ultimate love-on for ourselves begins with what passes through our lips on a daily basis. Taking extreme self-care requires us to take a good, hard look at our emotional connection with food.

It's not only WHAT we eat. It's WHY we are eating that holds the real key to transforming our bodies and our lives.

TRUTH: We don't eat just for fuel. Often we eat to soothe hurt feelings or stuff pains and wounds that make us feel yucky.

Are you in on this? I know I am.

Sure, I'm fit, but that doesn't mean I haven't gone through the same struggles my clients and listeners have gone through. I get it. Really, I do. I can remember the self-loathing and the food battles like they were yesterday, if I *choose* to.

And that is the truth. I have made different *choices* for myself.

So can you.

Personally, a huge part of the reason why preparing for a Bikini Fitness Competition is so challenging is exactly this: I have to face full-on my patterns of how I use food as reward, and even more important, how I use food to cope. And I am telling you, this process to self-awareness ain't always pretty! Ha!

No longer using food as a "source to soothe," I am forced to deal head-on with any unresolved issues in my life, and the process can be painful. Okay, not "can be" – IS.

But just like a monk goes into silent retreat or an athlete prepares for a big competition, he or she understands that the journey starts and ends within. This is no different for you and me as we embrace living a more healthy and fit lifestyle.

Honestly, it would be so much easier if it was just that easy to say, "Hey, I'm going to lose 10 pounds," and we just did it. The truth is that we shed way more than the physical weight when we embrace a lifestyle transformation. Old patterns and behaviors, like old luggage we haul behind us, have to be kicked to, *and* left at, the curb.

Through any transformation, our personal issues, past hurts and feelings of rejection, fear, and loneliness rear their ugly heads! This part of the INNER FIT SELF REBIRTH is not always easy, but so worth it. You have to trust me on this one.

Will you? Please say YES. I so have your back!

So why do many of us experience epic fails on our health goals? One word: FEAR! Fear of failure! Fear of success. Fear of letting go. Fear of judgment. Fear of the unknown. Fear of… you name it!

Our fear and resistance to face the music of our pasts are often the real causes of diet failures and exercise plans getting waylaid. Our commitment falls away when our "ugly" rears its head.

Letting Go: Kissing Goodbye to What No Longer Serves You!

"Help! I want to let go, but I don't know where to start!"

When we decide to move fully into our process of transformation and begin to embrace our Inner Hottie, often the relationships around us, as well as the relationship with ourselves, suddenly look like they need a whole lotta spit-polishing! For real!

What are you tolerating in your life that has to go – person, place, thing, behavior? You gotta name it and deal with it. It is time to reframe your life by releasing self-sabotaging language, thoughts, and behaviors. This time is long overdue.

And the benefits of having tolerations resolved?

Delicious and yummy freedom from self-sabotage, self-loathing, and any of those other crappy and self-defeating ways of being that you are ready and willing (please say you are ready and willing!) to kick to the proverbial curb.

Please review the previous chapter on tolerations, and be sure some of the things on the list include releasing your patterns or behaviors around emotional eating.

If they are not on there yet, go ahead and add them to the list. You are just going to love crossing these off in the not-too-distant future for sure, so be ready for some giddy excitement when that day comes. And it will!

The Setting Yourself Free from Emotional Eating Action Plan

- What does food mean to you? Please fill in the space with as many adjectives or nouns as you can come up with.
     Food is...

- What changes in your diet are you ready to embrace to release the weight that no longer serves you?

- What self-sabotaging behavior are you ready to let go of?

- Please write below the new eating habits and behavior changes you now embrace that will allow you to unleash your fit self to the nth degree! You got this!

_____
_____
_____
_____

My Living Sexy Fit Freedom from Emotional Eating Manifesto!

Today I, _____, am ready to release
_____
_____
_____

I know that this behavior no longer serves me. I will take the following action,
_____
_____
_____
_____, so that I can release my sexy fit self and attain the body I desire, the lifestyle that reflects who I am, and the peace that I deserve – because I am worthy!

Lovingly signed by:

_____

Please post your Living Sexy Fit Freedom from Emotional Eating Manifesto or carry it with you so you can read it out loud three times in a row, two times a day, preferably when you wake up and when you go to bed each day, until you are living it all out every day!

Bravo for taking this brave first step! You are amazing!

Kate's Love Note to you beautiful peeps who struggle with food bingeing, anorexia, or any other ways so many of us use food to quell our sorrow, anger, loneliness, or dead-on grief: You are not alone. You deserve more. You are worthy of self-love and self-acceptance.

Really.

You are.

Reach out to a coach or therapist who can help you face your emotions so you can be free to soar. The world awaits your brilliance.

OK, so let's dig into the Living Sexy Fit nutritional nuggets,

shall we? ☺

CHAPTER 13

The Living Sexy Fit Clean Eats Lifestyle – *Nutritional Mojo*

"CAN'T I JUST DO THE TREADMILL AND BE DONE?"

So many of us are under the illusion that all we have to do to get in shape and look sizzling-hot like Beyonce is to get on the treadmill and maybe cut out a couple of our fast-food runs.

Well, I am here to burst that bubble, and quick.

Are you ready?

From my experience, your nutrition, not exercise, is 70% of the Living Sexy Fit game!

"EEK," I hear you scream! "This cannot be! I was just born fat, my whole family is overweight, my husband makes me eat it, my metabolism is just slow. My extra weight is not anything to do with my nutrition!" Blah, blah, blah...

Sorry, I am not buying <u>any</u> of it.

Clean eating is the pathway to your fitness paradise. In order to live the Sexy Fit Lifestyle, you have to be all in on cleaning up your nutrition so you can gain the quickest benefits and regain the vitality and sizzle you long for.

"But wait, Kate, what about the other 30%?"

Great question.

From my experience, the other 30% can be divided into the following:

     20% exercise
     10% genetics

I know. Pick your jaw up off the floor.

All I am going to give you is 10% credit toward your genetics??

Yup, sorry about that, too.

Okay, so now that we have cleared that up, let's dig in to why your nutrition plays such a crucial role, and then we will talk about how we can use exercise to put your sexy machine into overdrive.

So, believe it or not, the odds of nature are actually *stacked in your favor* – and not vice versa.

This is worth repeating: The odds of nature are actually stacked in your favor, *if* you are ready to make adjustments to what, when, and how you eat.

For some of you, this may be a small shift. For others, this may be a much bigger change-up. I get this. But what is more important is how big the desire is to manifest your best self, who is just waiting to be unleashed.

You have the power and strength to unleash the powerful and magnificent person that lies within using the right and proper action plan that will be just right for *you*, designed by *you*!

By applying the **Clean Eats Action Plan** and embracing the exercises in this book, you can peg the red on your hotness odometer. I look forward to helping.

So to review, in order to live the Sexy Fit Lifestyle, you must adopt the "EAT CLEAN and Get Fit" Game Plan, which includes:

- Eating all kinds of yummy foods that flip on your fat-burning pilot and convert your body from a fat-manufacturing machine to a fat-burning machine.

- Incorporate strength training into your regime to increase your muscle mass for increased fat-burning power.

- Include a moderate cardiovascular exercise program that will round out your full body renovation!

If weight loss is your goal, jump in and feel confident that you will lose the weight at a rate of 1 to 2 pounds per week as a result of adopting the **Eat Clean and Get Fit Lifestyle.**

Think about it: In 28 days you could be 5 to 10 pounds lighter, increase your fat-burning muscle significantly and experience greater energy and sex appeal!

How amazing will that be??

"Celebrate each and every success you experience.

Don't wait for someone else to celebrate for you."
"Let the celebration come from within!"

Listen, I am the first one to admit that I love food. I also love how food—the preparing it, the sharing of it—is one of the most beautiful opportunities for us to be in community with the people we love and care for.

One of my greatest pleasures in life is making awesome meals for my kids and friends. Food is nurturing. It shows our caring and our generosity and love.

Unfortunately, the sad truth is that two out of three people in America are overweight or obese, and the problem is only getting worse. We have gone from viewing food as celebration to using it now as a way to soothe and satiate all kinds of emotional and biological impulses that have been thrown all out of whack from how and what we have been eating.

It is clear that the "quick fix, get skinny" diet culture we live in is *not* working. We need to shift our fundamental ways of thinking, believing, and ACTING to create a culture that is healthy and fit *from the inside out.*

The 80/20 Rule of the Living Sexy Fit Lifestyle

This is why I would like to introduce to you the 80/20 rule of Living Sexy Fit. If you imagine each day focusing on your nutrition, I would like you to see at least 80% of your food choices coming from the Clean Eats Macronutrients listed in the following chapter. The remaining 20% can be choices made from perhaps not the most clean of foods.

Now that does *not* mean 10 Oreos, an extra grande latte with extra cream and sugar, a fried platter with all the fixings. What I am speaking of is perhaps two cookies, a latte with milk and a small shot of whipped cream, a piece of broiled haddock with a baked potato and a teaspoon of sour cream (plain Greek yogurt is a great substitute for sour cream, by the way).

You see, you can still enjoy the flavors and foods you love and crave. But accept that the portions must be smaller. They will be just a sampling of what was once a bloodbath of calorie consumption every day.

For example, say your calorie allotment for the day is 1,500 calories. 80% of that is 1,200, so your treat for the day would be a yummy of no more than 300 calories.

Take back your ability to savor your food. It is your right to find enjoyment in what you eat. And I promise you, as you clean up your food choices, your desire to binge on junk and your craving for unhealthy food will fall by the wayside.

Adopting the Living Sexy Fit 80/20 rule, you'll not only be happier by how you look and feel but also hotter than you ever felt, because there's nothing that kills your sexy like excess junk in your trunk!

If you slip up, and have too much of something that you know wasn't feeding your white hot sizzle, relax! One bad meal is no reason to send you into a tailspin of despair and self-loathing.

You have the ability to *course-correct* one meal at a time; embrace self-love and clean eats, and be prepared to see how your relationship with food becomes once again an experience of celebration.

Remember: You have the ability and the power to course-correct after a "cheat meal" or a binge that did not fuel or soothe your soul.

What's done is done.

Jump on the clean eating track at the next meal. That's it! One binge does not define you. You are here to live in your magnificence! Focus on the amazing vision you have created for yourself and call out loud, "Next!"

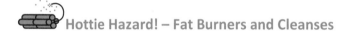 **Hottie Hazard! – Fat Burners and Cleanses**

I am frequently asked my opinion on the latest fat-burning cleanse or other newfangled diet regimen. My answer is <u>always</u> the same:

> There is no better Rx than eating clean, exercising your body, hydrating, and living in peace and self-love and acceptance. The Living Sexy Fit lifestyle is a way of life that no pill or diet can replace. Embracing the LSF lifestyle is about letting go of the fear and need for the quick fix, and realizing that you already possess everything you need.

CHAPTER 14

The Living Sexy Fit Clean Eats System – *Choosing Foods That Fuel the Machine!*

As I'm a breakthrough coach, fitness guru, and bikini competitor, everyone wants to know my secret weapon to a leaner and fitter physique. They want to know what exercise will rid them of their bellies or their thighs so they can look and feel lean and vibrant.

If there is a secret weapon, it is not doing the latest core training, spending hours on the elliptical, or doing hot yoga three times a day. Instead, it's creating a sound nutritional plan that will allow you to shed extra weight and live a life with more energy and vitality.

Ultimately, isn't this what we are all looking for?

It's important that we go over some basic nutrition information so you are clear on what healthy foods you will eat on the Living Sexy Fit Clean Eats Lifestyle Plan.

Let's start by reviewing the big three yummos – macronutrients.

MACRONUTRIENTS: proteins, carbs and healthy fats – all the goodness that supplies our bodies what they need for energy and repair.

1. **PROTEIN** – Consuming a healthy dose of protein is essential in the Living Sexy Fit Clean Eats Plan. Protein builds muscle, stabilizes blood sugars, feeds muscle tissues, and revs up your metabolism.

   Excellent protein sources include the following:

   ✓ lean beef cuts
   ✓ chicken breast
   ✓ turkey breast
   ✓ ground turkey
   ✓ eggs/egg whites
   ✓ haddock
   ✓ cod
   ✓ halibut
   ✓ flounder
   ✓ salmon*
   ✓ swordfish*
   ✓ tuna*
   ✓ protein powder (whey or vegan)
   ✓ tofu
   ✓ tempeh

These foods also are excellent fat sources that can count toward your daily fat needs.

By increasing your protein intake, you will most likely experience an increased sense of being satiated between meals, increased stamina, decreased fatigue, and a noticeably leaner physique!

When I first increased my protein consumption when I made the shift in my diet years ago, the change in my physique was dramatic. My body fat dropped by several percentage points, and I felt stronger and more energetic throughout the day. I was amazed.

2. **CARBOHYDRATES**—two ways—choose wisely!

EEK! The dreaded carb!

There is so much carb-bashing in the media about they are the main culprit in our country's obesity epidemic. For years, our "war on carbs" saturated the market, instilling fear in millions and misinforming the multitudes.

So are carbs really that bad??

Well, yes and no.

As a society, our consumption of so much processed food has turned many of us into *carb junkies*. It is this processed crap that wreaks havoc on out metabolism and jacks up our insulin levels into the danger zone. This is the fuel behind our obesity epidemic and where we will all benefit from making the changes on reducing our consumption of crapola.

So, first I want to distinguish between the two classes of carbohydrates and how we consume the "good ones" on the Living Sexy Fit Clean Eats Plan.

When I'm talking about carbs in the LSF plan, I'm talking about the good carbs that fuel your hotness and keep your machine running clean all day long.

"But wait! How can we tell between a good carb and a bad carb?"

Great question.

Let's start with the principle behind low glycemic carbs and high glycemic carbs and how the body assimilates and breaks these down.

High glycemic carbs or simple carbs are converted to sugar pronto, jacking up insulin production and dousing your fat-burning capacity in a flash. These are not so great and need to be consumed at a minimum on the plan.

Examples of these dirty rotten culprits: *anything* with refined flour or sugar. Yup, all the white stuff filled with naughty sugars partnered with nasty fats that taste so good, but are like weapons of mass destruction to your hotness.

You know what I am talking about! All those "foods" that tempt our hotness factor and give us rot gut and drop our fat-burning capabilities to zero. If you cannot resist these stinkers, do not, I mean DO NOT, keep them in your house. They are extremely sneaky and know when to come in for the kill when your emotions are weak and your "hunger" is high.

Just say no! They are the trickiest, sneakiest devils you will ever meet, especially at the beginning of your Living Sexy Fit journey. Do not be tempted by their sugar sprinkle, sparkle, or tantalizing sales pitch. Slam the door, give them the back of your hand, and deny them at all costs.

It's hard. But it's possible.

You are here to do great things.

Do not forget it!

Moving on to the low glycemic foods, let's expand on these good carbs, those that jack up your love machine!
1. Good Carbs #1 – the stick-to-your-ribbers.
2. Good Carbs #2 – fresh and crunchy nibbles.

The Good Carb Stuff #1

Here's your LSF Good Carbs #1 list:

- ✓ oatmeal
- ✓ brown rice
- ✓ sweet potatoes
- ✓ yams

- ✓ rice cakes
- ✓ Ezekiel bread (sprouted wheat)
- ✓ whole grain pasta
- ✓ spaghetti squash
- ✓ pumpkin

The Good Carb Stuff #2

When we are talking Good Carbs #2, picture the rainbow, baby. Your shopping cart should be multicolored and bursting with color!

Munch and crunch on your veggies! Why are these so good for you? Because you can munch on these items to your heart's content (Within reason! Please, no broccoli bingeing!). Good Carbs #2 are filling, loaded with vitamins and minerals, and low in calories. They also slow down the absorption of your food, which boosts the fat-burning furnace. Yippee!

Think of fiber filled food as "nature's Brillo pad," giving your insides a good scrubbing. A clean system is a happy system. The high fiber content in these foods act like a magnet in your body as it travels through, hooking up with some junk so you will have less in your trunk.

How cool is that??

Eating clean allows your body to absorb more good and
slough off the bad so you can be spit-shined from the inside out.

Your veggie list:

- ✓ lettuce (all kinds, the darker the better)
- ✓ broccoli
- ✓ zucchini
- ✓ cauliflower
- ✓ spinach

- ✓ green beans
- ✓ asparagus
- ✓ peppers (red & green)
- ✓ kale
- ✓ onions
- ✓ mushrooms

Fresh veggies are best.

HARSH TRUTH: Fruits are treats in the Living Sexy Fit Lifestyle! Sure, fruits have fiber; however, they are loaded with sugars that can skyrocket your insulin levels. Limiting fruit servings to two per day keeps you in the red-hot sexy fit zone.

Your fruits list:

- ✓ grapefruit – ½
- ✓ berries (blue, rasp, straw, black) – ¼ cup small berries, ½ cup bigger berries
- ✓ apple – 1 small
- ✓ pear – 1 small
- ✓ banana – ½

> <u>Taste Buds Reboot</u> – Like any new habit, it can take two to three weeks for your taste buds and cravings to reset.

3. **FATS** – yes, fats! Hip, hip, hooray!

Just like when we're talking about carbs, there are some good fats and some not-so-good fats. In the LSF program, it's important to differentiate between the two.

Fat is essential for:

a. Energy. Gram for gram, fat is the best energy source. Fat provides 9 calories per gram. Carbs and proteins provide only 4 per gram.
b. Building healthy cell membranes for each and every part of your body including your brain. Without a healthy dose of good fat, your brain suffers and produces brain fog.
c. The absorption of important fat-soluble vitamins, including A, D, E and K.
d. Making hormones – and we need those suckers! They make up some of the most important substances in the body, including prostaglandins, hormonelike substances that regulate many of the body's functions.
e. Our skin, hair, and nails. We need fat to produce and keep our "lovelies" lovely.

The fats listed below contain essential fatty acids (EFA's), which our bodies don't make on their own and which play an important role in so many of our bodily functions, including healthy skin and happy muscles and joints.

Healthy fats:

- ✓ almond oil
- ✓ olive oil
- ✓ flaxseed oil
- ✓ fish/tuna oil
- ✓ nuts (almonds, cashews, walnuts)
- ✓ salmon
- ✓ avocados
- ✓ coconut oil
- ✓ walnut oil

And the bad fats? Say adios and farewell to animal fats and other heavily processed foods that are jacked up with trans-fatty acids that wreak havoc on your Living Sexy Fit Lifestyle Plan.

Those yuckos include all the whites, white sugar, white flour, fat-laden convenience foods and bakery goods and fast-food junk that will wreak havoc on your Hottie factor. A little taste is okay once in a while, but it is time to say adios and au revoir (Lawrence Welk style) to eating junk that only loads up your trunk.

Micronutrients

Vitamins and minerals serve an important role in regulating cell function, converting food into energy, and maintaining all biological functions. Personally, I am not a big proponent of popping pills. But, based on the fact that much of the produce we consume comes from heavily depleted soil, I believe it is a good idea to add a multivitamin-and-mineral supplement to your daily regimen. I also take a calcium supplement and vitamin D for strong and healthy bones.

Kate's Nutritional Tip:

I am a minimal supplements kind o' girl. However, because it is tough to eat perfectly, I supplement my diet with a healthy vitamin-and-mineral supplement with no fillers or sugars, and also with vitamin D for strong and healthy bones.

LIVING SEXY FIT CLEAN EATS SHOPPING LIST

PROTEIN	NON-STARCHY VEGETABLES	STARCHY VEGETABLES	FRUIT	GOOD FAT
Lean beef cuts	Lettuce	Oatmeal	Grapefruit	Almond oil
Chicken breast	Broccoli	Brown rice	Blueberries	Olive oil
Turkey breast	Zucchini	Sweet potatoes	Strawberries	Flaxseed oil
Ground turkey	Cauliflower	Yams	Raspberries	Fish/tuna oil
Eggs/egg whites	Spinach	Rice cakes	Blackberries	Almonds
Haddock	Green beans	Ezekiel bread	Apples	Cashews
Cod	Asparagus	Whole grain pasta	Pears	Walnuts
Halibut	Peppers	Spaghetti squash	Bananas	Salmon
Flounder	Kale	Pumpkin		Avocados
Salmon	Onions	Quinoa		Coconut oil
Swordfish	Mushrooms			Walnut oil
Tuna				
Protein powder				
Tofu				
Tempeh				

CHAPTER 15

The Living Sexy Fit Clean Eats System – *the Importance of Metabolism and Hydration!*

8 SUREFIRE WAYS TO SPEED UP YOUR METABOLISM!

What does metabolism mean anyway? Metabolism is the process by which food is broken down and converted into energy, which fuels your living sexy machine right down to the cellular level.

Often, people who excessively diet can sabotage their metabolism. However, the truth is that *very few people genetically have "slow metabolism."* You can speed up your metabolism by putting the following healthy habits into practice today:

1. Increase your muscle mass. People with higher levels of muscle tend to have a higher resting metabolic rate. That means you burn more calories just chilling out then less muscular folks do. Why? Muscle burns more calories than fat.

According to the American Council on Exercise (ACE), of which I am a Certified Personal Trainer, each pound of fat burns only 2 calories a day, while muscle burns between 35 and 50 calories per day. That is a significant difference. So go ahead with your resistance training today to build calorie-consuming muscle, increasing your metabolism as a result.

2. Focus on intensity in your cardio program. Doing sustained-level intensity is great, but performing a higher level of cardio (or HIIT training) will be more effective at increasing your metabolic rate. Examples of HIIT are a Spin class, a varied program on a treadmill or elliptical machine, and a jog workout of varying intensity for a minimum of 20 minutes to get your heart pumping and metabolism burning.

3. Embrace grazing. I know so many of our mothers told us to get out of the kitchen, stop snacking, and wait for dinner to eat. Studies show that eating more frequently each day keeps the metabolism elevated. As a result, you will burn more calories throughout the day, even at rest. Choose healthy lean proteins and vegetables as your primary meal sources, with moderate amounts of fruit and healthy fats to keep you going.

4. Eat more protein. This tip is what made the most significant difference to my lean physique. First, protein makes you feel full longer due to its dense makeup, reducing your need to binge on carbs to reach the same level of satiation. In addition, your body burns more calories to break down proteins (8 calories per gram for proteins vs. 4 for carbs). My clients hear this from me the most: "How is your protein level?" If you want a lean physique, your lean protein consumption must increase. Chicken, turkey, fish, and the occasional beef and pork are your best sources for increasing your metabolism and providing longer-lasting satiation.

Personally, I have not eaten beef or pork since I was 5 years old, however I find plenty of ways to get my protein in, by eating plenty of fish, chicken and turkey. I have lived a moe vegetarian diet, however, I personally feel stronger and have more energy and frankly, have a better physique based on what I believe is a richer protein diet.

Vegans take note: Those of you who are vegetarian have a greater challenge in balancing your protein to carb ratio, but it is possible with careful planning and proper education.

5. Eat your fiber! Higher-fiber foods (oatmeal, flaxseed, brown rice, sweet potatoes, asparagus, broccoli, green beans) provide steady, long-lasting energy and make you feel full and satisfied longer. And who doesn't love a big, ole' salad??

6. Drink up! Black coffee and green tea! A moderate amount of caffeine (1 to 2 cups a day) raises your metabolism slightly, increases concentration and improves heart health. Green tea also contains antioxidants that boost the immune system. Sip away!

7. Eat your healthy fats! Monounsaturated fats like olive oil help reduce cholesterol, triglycerides, and blood pressure. Polyunsaturated fats such as walnuts, almonds, flaxseeds, and salmon, are filled with omega-3s and reduce triglycerides and inflammation in the body. Coconut oil is an all over yummo. Plus it has also shown to kill off sugar cravings. Bring it in!

8. Stay hydrated. When the body does not have enough water, several functions slow down, including the ability to burn calories. Muscles are roughly 65% to 70% water, so if they are not fully hydrated, they cannot perform as effectively, thus decreasing your calorie burn. Also, the body is not as efficient at burning fat when it is not hydrated for down shifting your metabolism. Glug away!

How much water is enough is still open to debate, but one study found that adults who drink 8 or more glasses of water a day burned more calories than those who drank 4 or fewer glasses a day. Shoot for 50% of your body weight in ounces as your **base** target amount.

Your metabolism is not a life sentence! By applying the principles above, you can engage your overdrive for calorie-boosting delight!

Hydrate! Hydrate!

I know we just spoke about the importance of water consumption to boost your metabolism. I believe so strongly in keeping yourself hydrated that I feel it necessary to pontificate just a little bit more. ☺

Did you know that water makes up 60% to 70% of your body? Wow! Recent studies show that staying hydrated plays an important role in boosting your metabolism, which fuels your calorie-burning machine.

Proper hydration does the following:

- increases heart rate
- boosts metabolism
- increases the efficiency of your energy systems
- decreases appetite
- helps regulate appetite
- dilutes sodium retention which prevents bloating
- promotes healthy skin, your biggest organ
- increases blood volume so more oxygen gets into muscles

Dehydration – "Deprivation of vitality." EEK!

Water helps deliver nutrients to our organs and tissues, and helps in the removal of toxins and waste from the body. It also helps regulate body temperature.

Dehydration causes the following:

- increased wrinkles
- bags under the eyes
- headaches
- chapped lips
- constipation
- lethargy
- mood swings
- metabolism boosts of approximately 3%

Doesn't reading this make you thirsty? I'm thirsty just writing about it! Go ahead and take a break in your reading and drink a quick 8ozs. Your body will thank you.

More on Clean Eats ahead. Don't miss it!

To sign up for Kate's free newsletter for more fitness and wellness tips, go to www.kate-mckay.com/freenewsletter

Living Sexy Fit   by Kate McKay

CHAPTER 16

The Living Sexy Fit Clean Eats Playbook

OK, so now it's time to move on to some more of the nuts and bolts of the Living Sexy Fit Clean Eats Plan, including how much to eat and how often.

Nutritional Know-How Tidbits

"How do I know how much to eat to attain my Living Sexy Fit goals?"

Hey, check this out! As people have different goals based on their starting point and overall health, it is important that you visit a doctor, a reputable nutritionist, or a trainer who has a high level of nutritional knowledge to set a calorie range for you that will most benefit your individual goals.

A simple rule of thumb: Your daily calorie requirement is roughly 10 calories per pound of body weight. If you are looking to lose weight, base that amount on your ideal realistic target weight. If you are an athlete, the calorie requirement will be significantly higher. Again, please speak to your doctor or nutritionist to ensure what would be your daily calorie target based on your goals.

Some important facts on macronutrients, and rough targets to shoot for:

Protein:

½ gram to 1 gram of protein per 1 lb. of body weight per day
4 calories per gram
Protein size that fits in your palm, 3 to 4 oz. per serving

Carbs:

½ to 1½ grams of carbs per 1 lb. of body weight
4 calories per gram
Fist size is a serving. Green veggies are the best bang for your buck.

Fats:

2-3 tablespoons of fat a day 9 calories per gram

Suggestions: Add 1 tablespoon of oil to your salad or veggies and you've got your fat calories covered. A tablespoon of coconut oil in your oatmeal, delish.

Let's chat about portion control, the biggest Living Sexy Fit saboteur. Please refer to the chart below. When we truly see a visual cue on how much we should be eating, compared with what we currently consume, this can come as a terrible shock.

Hand Measurement	Foods	Calories (approx.)
Fist – 1 cup	Brown rice, sweet potato	200
	Fruit	150
	Veggies	40
Palm – 3 oz.	Meat	160
	Fish	160
	Poultry	160
Handful – 1 oz.	Nuts	170
	Raisins	85
2 Handfuls – 1 oz.	Chips	150
	Popcorn	120
	Pretzels	100
Thumb-size – 1 oz.	Peanut butter	170
	Hard cheese	100
Thumbnail- 1 tsp.	Cooking oil	40
	Butter	35

Tricks I suggest to adjust to eating smaller and healthier portions:

1. Drink a big glass of water before you eat. I drink room temperature water because I can drink it more easily.
2. Use a small salad plate or soup bowl to eat your meals.
3. Use juice glasses (6 to 8 oz.) to drink anything besides water.
4. Say goodbye to mindless eating. Concentrate on what you are eating and savor the flavors of your healthy foods. Turn off the tube!
5. Use baby spoons to eat dessert. It really makes you savor every bite.
6. Make a big batch of protein and veggie soup at least once a week.
7. Get adequate rest. A well-rested body tames bingeing.
8. Keep the junk out of the house if you know you cannot resist. Why put yourself through the torture?
9. Eat 3 oz. of protein before you go out to socialize to prevent overeating.

MEAL PLANNING FREQUENCY ON THE LSF PLAN:

Are you ready? This is it, Baby! The ticket to having the body of your dreams!

- Eat!
- Eat More of the Good Stuff!
- Eat Less of the Bad Stuff!
- Eat Clean at Least 80% of the Time!
- Eat More Often!

Yes! 5 times a day, every 2½ to 3 hours a day, is a must to get the body of your dreams and the energy and vitality you've only dreamed of!

Here's how the math works:

- 1,200 calories a day/5 = 240 calories per meal

- 1,600 calories a day/5 = 320 calories per meal

- 1,800 calories a day/5 = 360 calories per meal

- 2,000 calories a day/5 = 400 calories per meal

"So what IS a calorie?"

A calorie is a unit of measurement that represents the energy value of food. It's how we measure how much energy it takes our bodies to break down food.

In order for you to avoid a calorie dump, eating more frequently is a must. Say goodbye to calorie dumping! Continued fuel prevents insulin from skyrocketing, fat cells from plumping, and energy levels from crashing through the floor.

Be kind to your body by taking care of it lovingly. Your body doesn't deserve to be calorie-deprived, dumped on, binged, purged, and mistreated. Love on this beautiful vessel, your portal to peace, freedom, and living a sexy fit life.

You deserve it. You are ready to embrace this level of self-care.

"What's happening to me?? I feel like a hot mess!"

Aah! Hormones. Insulin levels. Withdrawal from toxins and toxic junk. The first week can be a little rough. Plan on it! Journal, hydrate, exercise, talk to your accountability partner. As you move through your Living Sexy Fit transformation, understand that often your emotions will wreak havoc as you release old eating habits. Infilling this void with self-love and extreme self-care, and deepening relationships with people who support and understand what you are going through, are essential.

And remember, this too shall pass. Your hotness awaits, so stay on task and keep your vision alive and brewing.

HOW TO "CHEAT" ON THE LSF PROGRAM

"Cheater! Cheater! Pumpkin Eater!"

First, I want to revisit the 80/20 rule. To really get the greatest effect, you must embrace clean eating 80% of the time.

- 80% to 90% food for fuel.

- 10% to 20% food for enjoyment (within reason – Two cookies, not six. A small iced coffee with cream, not an extra-large mocha frappe). You gotta' redefine a treat! A treat is NOT a sleeve of Girl Scout cookies!

Plan in a couple cheat meals a week. A cheat meal is not an all-you-can-eat smorgasbord. However, if you have a hankering, enjoy one of your favs not on the Clean Eats List. Remember: it is all about portion control. Savor your food and got back on the clean eats train on your next meal. That's it!

You can do it!

Clean Eats Daily Planner

Meal Time example:
> Breakfast: 7 a.m.
> Mini: 10 a.m.
> Lunch: 1 p.m.
> Mini: 4 p.m.
> Dinner: 6 p.m.
> Optional Mini: 8:30 p.m.

Kate's Daily Sampling on Her Clean Eats Meal Plan Example

Meal 1
> ¼ cup dry oatmeal
> 3 eggs (1 yolk, 3 egg whites)
> or a protein smoothie with protein powder
> ¼ cup blueberries and almond milk w coconut oil

Meal 2
> 12 almonds
> 1 apple or ground turkey with green beans and ½ cup brown rice

Meal 3
> Ground chicken, turkey, beef on greens, red pepper, 4 oz. sweet or brown rice

Meal 4
> Rice cake with 1 tsp. almond butter or unsweetened Greek yogurt with honey and 12 almonds

Meal 5

Fish or chicken with broccoli and greens with healthy oil dressing or Chicken with green beans or asparagus   or... protein shake with almond milk and protein powder

Feel free, if you are not totally famished after 2½ to 3 hours, to make the next meal slightly smaller – but whatever you do, please don't skip! Your metabolism will go on slo-mo!

Important: Muscles are <u>metabolically active tissue,</u> which means they use all kinds of calories to keep them all moving and grooving. Muscles are their own fat-burning, calorie-churning machine. The more muscle you have, the hotter and more efficiently you burn. And THAT is a good thing!

PORTION CONTROL

What Your Plate Should Look Like:

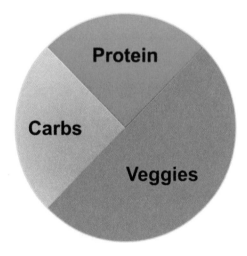

What your plate should not look like:

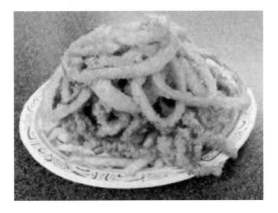

Kate's Fit Tip: Use smaller plates to help with portion control – and stay away from red dishes. Studies show you will eat more on red! Yikes!

Clean Eats Food Preparation:
The Ticket to Your Living Sexy Fit Success!

A good offense beats the best defense. Food preparation on the Living Sexy Fit Program is essential. I spend an hour three times a week preparing my meals for the days in between and portioning them in containers so I can just grab and go when I leave the house.

Not having the time is not an excuse. If you want to have that sexy sizzle, then your food prep time is a must. Plan it around other activities, invite your family to help, play great music, listen to an audio program, but please commit to this crucial step.

The cleanest fuel of all – self-love and self-acceptance.

You got this.

Living Sexy Fit Clean Eats Summary:

1. Eat More – five meals each day.
2. Eat Breakfast – make this meal non-negotiable. Eat within an hour of rising.
3. Eat Protein with Every Meal – eating a lean protein and a complex carbohydrate at every meal prolongs digestion and encourages stable blood sugars.
4. Eat Healthy Fats – Eat two to three servings of healthy fats every day.
5. Know Your Portion Sizes.
6. Prepare Your Meals in Advance – meal preparation is essential for ultimate success.
7. Drink Water/Stay Hydrated – drink no less than 64 ounces of water a day.

Clean Eats + Smaller Plates + Body Moving and Grooving = Hotness!

You Got This!!

Remember: Not being properly hydrated causes your metabolism to slow down, meaning you are putting your fat-burning machine on simmer. Glug up the water for furnace-boosting power!

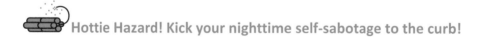 **Hottie Hazard! Kick your nighttime self-sabotage to the curb!**

When is the primary time that diet self-sabotage is most likely to occur? At night, when defenses are low!

Avoid the Living Sexy Fit saboteur by taking immediate action to put this nasty habit to bed once and for all!

1. Clean out your cabinets! The best offense against this habit is to adopt a great defense – dump the junk! Clear out the refrigerator and cabinets of food that you know will lead to a binge. Not only will you benefit, but so will your entire family.

   My last junk eats sweep included stale crackers, chocolate peanut butter spread, Oreos, a can of pineapple in heavy syrup, a packet of Equal, and chocolate from last Christmas. Oh my!

   Action: Grab a garbage bag and go at this one. It is easy and a quick fix to prevent future diet sabotage.

2. Cut back on tube time! Increased TV/screen time has a direct correlation with a bigger waistline, whether it is due to lack of activity, increased mindless eating, or increased commercial watching leading to junk-food brain programming. Beware!

   Choose a couple of shows you enjoy, and then turn off the tube as soon as they are over.

   Whatever you do, do not eat your primary meals in front of the tube. Be present when you eat. Learn to savor the food you consume and the company you keep for greater quality of life all around.

   Turn off the TV and find something else to fill your background noise. Try classical music or silence to create a background to your life. Envision how your life will be when you are at your ideal weight and living an active and fit lifestyle.

3. Dress for success! Choose one piece of exercise/workout wear to put on under your clothes as a continual reminder that you will work out at some time during your day. I always wear an exercise shirt under my dress shirt so that I am ready to go and don't come up with some lame excuse to blow off the gym. My commitment to the best me is way more important. Stay committed to the best YOU!

CHAPTER 17

Recipes for the Living Sexy Fit Lifestyle

Breakfast

<u>Eggs, Eggs and More Eggs!</u>
3 or 4 hardboiled eggs without the yolks
Mix your egg whites with the following suggested seasonings:
- Mrs. Dash spices (any variety)
- fresh herbs
- hot sauce
- a sprinkle of Parmesan cheese

<u>Oatmeal Suggestions</u>
- ¼ cup dried with water and ¼ cup frozen blueberries. Microwave for 130 seconds.
- ¼ cup dried with water. Microwave and serve with a sprinkle of slivered almonds or 4 to 5 walnut halves.
- ¼ cup oatmeal with water. Microwave with water for 130 seconds. Top with a heaping teaspoon of coconut oil and ½ teaspoon of coconut sugar.

Veggie-Eggy Bake

Spray a medium pan with oil or a couple drops of oil and lightly sauté ¼ onion and a small zucchini. Pour ½ cup of egg whites over the veggies and cook until the eggs start to set. Sprinkle with herbs and ½ teaspoon of Parmesan cheese. Place under the broiler until it's set and lightly brown. Serves two.

All-in-One Yummo
- ½ cooked sweet potato, sliced thinly
- 1 cup fresh spinach
- ¼ cup raspberries
- 1 tsp. cinnamon
- 1 tbsp. coconut oil
- ¼ cup of egg whites or 4 egg whites

Lightly sauté the sweet potato with a splash of cooking spray. Place the rest of the ingredients in the pan, starting with the coconut oil, and cook slowly until the egg has set.

Jessie's Protein Pancakes
- 1 scoop vanilla protein powder
- 1 tbsp. coconut flour
- ¼ cup oats
- 1 tbsp. psyllium husk (makes them fluffy)
- 1 tsp. baking soda
- dash of butter extract
- dash of coconut extract

Mix the ingredients and cook in a pan with a dash of coconut oil. Optional: Serve with protein pancake frosting.

Pancake Frosting
- 1 small tub of coconut milk yogurt
- ¼ teas of vanilla flavoring

Mix the vanilla into the yogurt. Put it in the fridge for an hour or overnight.

Michelle's Butterscotch Pancakes
- 4 oz. cooked sweet potato
- ½ scoop vanilla protein powder
- 3 to 4 drops butterscotch extract
- 3 extra-large eggs (no yolks)
- all-natural peanut butter
- splash of almond milk

Blend the ingredients. Pour slowly onto an oiled and heated pan, flip when bubbling, and enjoy! Makes 5 pancakes. 1-2 servings

Chocolate-Apple Crunch
- ½ cup chopped frozen apple
- ¼ cup oatmeal
- 1 scoop chocolate whey protein isolate
- 1 cup water
- ice

Put in a Blender and blend away!

Lunch/Dinner

Kathy's Open Face Bell Peppers
- 3 peppers
- ½ chopped onion
- ½ cup spinach
- 1 tbsp. olive oil
- 1 lb. ground chicken or turkey
- garlic salt
- Montreal chicken seasoning
- salt and pepper

Cut the peppers in half. Mix the onion, spinach, olive oil, and meat. Seasoning with the remaining ingredients. Fill the peppers with the stuffing and bake for 35 to 40 minutes at 375°F.

Amy's Anytime Tuna Lettuce Wraps
- romaine lettuce leaves
- canned/pouched tuna fish in water
- onions, peppers, celery
- squeeze of lemon juice
- mustard

Mix the tuna and ingredients that follow, and fill the leaves to your liking!

Crunch and Munch Lettuce Wraps
- 4 oz cooked ground turkey
- ½ steamed green beans
- ¼ avocado
- 1/8 c kidney beans
- salsa
- lettuce wraps

Mix the first five ingredients and fill the lettuce wraps. Yum!

Amanda's Keeping It Real Strawberry Salad
- 1 cup mixed greens
- ¼ cup strawberries
- 1½ tbsp. almonds
- mustard
- 4 oz. ground turkey or chicken

Kate's Chicken Salad Supreme
- 2 cooked boneless chicken breast
- ½ avocado
- pinch of sea salt and dash of fresh ground pepper
- 1 cup of mixed green lettuce
- 1-2 T of Balsamic dressing

Mix the first three ingredients. Serve on a piece of toasted Ezekiel bread, if you desire. Makes 2 to 3 servings.

Crunch Cranberry Chicken Salad
- 1 lb. chicken breast
- ½ cup chopped yellow onion
- 1/4 cup chopped celery
- 1/8 cup walnuts or pecans
- 1/8 cup dried cranberries
- 1/4 cup Greek yogurt
- 2 T Dijon mustard

Preheat an oven to 350°F. Cook the chicken breast on a foil-lined cookie sheet for 35 to 45 minutes. Let the chicken cool completely. While the chicken is cooking, finely chop the onion and celery. Add the chopped chicken, onion, celery, walnuts, cranberries, Greek yogurt, and Dijon mustard in a large bowl and mix until combined. Serve immediately or put in refrigerator to keep cool. Approx. 8 servings.

Janelle's Special Wonder!
- 8 oz. extra lean ground turkey
- 1 cup pure pumpkin
- ½ cinnamon
- 1 tsp. coconut oil

Preheat oven to 375°F. Cook the turkey in a pan with the coconut oil, then place it in a glass cooking dish or tin pan. Layer the turkey with a can of pumpkin. Cook for 20 minutes. Drizzle coconut and cinnamon on top. Serves 4.

Afternoon Pick Me Up Smoothie!
Organic yogurt and all-natural peanut butter give this snack a real protein boost.
- 1/2 cup almond milk
- 1/2 cup water
- 4 oz. plain nonfat yogurt
- 1 tbsp. natural peanut butter
- 3 fresh dates, pitted and chopped
- 1 tsp coconut oil

Place all of the ingredients together in a blender and puree until completely blended. This is better if it is not strained.

Mediterranean Chicken Salad
- 8 oz. chicken breast, sliced
- ¼ c green olives
- 1/8 c black olives
- balsamic vinegar
- Olive Oil
- Black Pepper
- Lemon squeeze
- 3 c mixed greens

Mix together first 7 ingredients and serve over greens. 2 servings

Diana's Low Carb Turkey Burger
- 2 portabella mushroom caps
- 4 oz. lean ground turkey, cooked
- 1 cup sautéed spinach in olive oil
- ⅛ cup chopped red onion
- spicy honey mustard

Lightly sauté the portabella mushrooms in a splash of olive oil. Remove mushrooms and add spinach. Fill mushroom with remaining ingredients and enjoy!

Pizza Pie-Moola My!
- 1 Food for Life Tortilla
- ⅛ cup marinara sauce
- 1 chicken sausage, cooked and sliced
- ¼ cup cottage cheese
- ½ cup baby spinach
- 2 to 3 slices fresh tomato

Cook right on a skillet until crispy!

Amy's Satisfy Your Fine Self Salmon

- ½ cup quinoa seasoned with Mrs Dash spice of your choice
- 4 oz. seared salmon
- 1 cup steamed spinach

Just a simple example of a deliciously balanced dish of good fats, starch, protein, and veggie.

Kate's Meatballs on the Go!

- 1 lb. lean ground turkey or extra lean beef
- ½ cup chopped red or white onions
- ½ cup chopped red peppers
- 1-2 t mustard (reg or honey mustard)
- ½ fresh squeezed lemon
- salt & pepper

Mix all ingredients together. Use a spoon to form the meatball and bake for 25 minutes at 350°F. Great for a meal on the go.

Diana's Low Carb, High Satisfaction Dinner Dish

- 1 cup snap peas
- ¼ cup mushrooms
- ½ red peppers, chopped
- 4 oz. salmon

Sauté peas and mushrooms in coconut oil, olive oil or avocado oil, and spice to your liking. Pan-sear the salmon, add the sugar snap peas.

Magical Maple Cinnamon Chicken

- 10-12 oz chicken, raw
- 1 teas maple extract
- 1 teas cinnamon
- ½ teas nutmeg

Mix maple extract, cinnamon, and nutmeg – just enough to mix and coat the chicken. Coat both sides, then bake at 350°F for 25 minutes in a lightly oiled pan (olive or coconut oil).

So good, you will be amazed!

Lemon-Broiled Swordfish

- 1 lb. swordfish steaks
- 2 tbsp. lemon juice
- 2 tbsp. water or dry white wine, or combination of both
- 1 tbsp. reduced salt soy sauce
- 2 cloves garlic, minced
- ¼ tsp. each dried parsley, basil, dill and marjoram
- ¼ tsp. black pepper
- cooking spray

Place the swordfish in a baking dish coated with low-fat cooking spray. Combine the remaining ingredients in a small bowl. Pour marinade over the swordfish and allow it to marinate for 30 to 40 minutes. Broil the fish for five minutes on each side or until the fish flakes easily. Use any remaining marinade to baste the fish while broiling. Makes 4 servings.

Roasted Sweet Potato Wedges #1

- 3 sweet potatoes
- cooking spray
- ½ tsp. chili powder
- ¼ tsp. salt
- ¼ tsp. cayenne pepper

Roasted Sweet Potato Wedges # 2

- Instead of cooking spray, coat in 1-2 teas coconut oil, sprinkle with cinnamon instead of chili powder, salt and cayenne pepper.

Preheat the oven to 400°F. Scrub the sweet potatoes well, trimming off any loose fibers. Cut into 1-inch wedges. Place the sweet potatoes in a single layer on a baking sheet sprayed with cooking spray. Lightly mist the potato wedges with cooking spray. Sprinkle the seasonings over the potatoes. Roast the potatoes in the oven for about 35 minutes, stirring occasionally. Sweet potatoes bake more quickly than regular potatoes, so make sure to check them often. Makes 4 servings.

Shrimp Quinoa Spinach Salad

Note: This recipe requires extra time to season and defrost the shrimp. If you didn't plan ahead, skip the seasonings and just place the shrimp in a colander under cold running water to defrost them more quickly.

- 8 oz. shrimp, precooked
- garlic salt
- Italian seasoning
- ½ cup water
- ¼ cup dry quinoa
- 1 tbsp. red wine vinegar
- 1 tsp. olive oil
- 2 cups fresh spinach leaves

Place the shrimp in a zip-top plastic bag and sprinkle liberally with garlic salt and Italian seasoning. Close the bag tightly and shake gently to spread spices throughout. Lay it flat in the refrigerator for two hours or until the shrimp have thawed. Bring the water and quinoa to a boil in a small saucepan over high heat. In a small bowl, whisk together the vinegar and olive oil. Arrange the spinach on a plate, spread the quinoa over the top, then add shrimp and dressing. Serves 2-3.

Steak Salad with Arugula, Lemon, Olive Oil, and Parmesan

- 8 oz. filet mignon, sliced in half
- kosher salt and cracked black pepper
- 4 small handfuls arugula
- juice of 1 lemon
- 1 tbsp. Olive Oil
- ½ oz. (a small dash) shaved Parmesan cheese
- nonstick cooking spray

Heat a grill to high and lightly coat it with nonstick cooking spray. Season the steak with salt and pepper, and grill to desired doneness. Toss the arugula with lemon juice and olive oil, and season with salt and pepper. Slice the steak and place it on top of the salad. Garnish with Parmesan cheese. Serve immediately. Serves 2.

Spinach Salad with Kale, Raspberries, and Grilled Chicken
- 1 tbsp. balsamic vinegar
- 1 tbsp. honey
- 1 garlic clove
- 4 basil leaves
- 2 tbsp. water
- 2 tbsp. extra-virgin olive oil
- kosher salt and cracked black pepper
- 2 cups baby spinach
- 1 to 2 cups kale
- ½ raspberries
- 8 oz. grilled chicken, sliced very thin

In a blender, puree the vinegar, honey, garlic, basil, and water. While pureeing, slowly add olive oil, salt, and pepper. (This will make extra dressing.) Toss the spinach, kale, strawberries, and chicken with 1 to 2 tablespoons of dressing. Serve immediately. Serves 2.

Snacks

Snack Basket

Sometimes we just want to munch on something. In between meals or after you have eaten everything for the day, it is important to have these snacks cut and ready for munching. Prepare them in individual ziplocs so you can grab and go.
- cucumber
- green pepper
- celery
- red peppers, green peppers

Other snacks on the go:
- One small apple with a sprinkle of cinnamon and a teaspoon of almond butter.

- Almonds (8 to 12 almonds) mixed with organic dark chocolate chips (12 to 15 chips).
- Hard boiled eggs on the fly with a small pear

Crunchy, Munchy Kale Chips
- 2-3 c kale
- 1 Tablespoon Coconut Oil
- Dash salt and pepper

Chop the kale, drizzle with coconut oil, and season. Cook at 325°F until crispy.

Treats

Sweet and Salty Yummo
- 1/8 c rolled oats
- 4 oz greek yogurt
- ¼ c blueberries
- ¼ t cinnamon
- Sprinkle chia seeds and pecans

Oatmeal Chocolate Delight
- ¼ cup oats
- 2/3 cup water
- ½ scoop chocolate protein powder
- 1 tsp. coconut oil

Microwave the oats for 90 seconds. Add ½ scoop of chocolate protein powder and 1 teaspoon of coconut oil. Delish!

Protein Bread Pudding
- 1 cup cooked brown rice
- 2 teas cocoa powder
- 1-2 scoops of protein powder

- 1 cup water or almond milk
- raspberries for a topping

Mix and eat hot or cold!

PART FOUR

The Living Sexy Fit

Buff Body Plan

CHAPTER 18

The Living Sexy Fit Buff Body Bootie Shake – *You Gotta' Move It, Move It!*

Working out—even that phrase doesn't sound fun to the majority of people! What we need is a reframe, a re-languaging—how about, PLAYING-OUT?!

Now I bring this up only partially in jest because ultimately the fastest way to celebrating your Living Sexy Fit self is to find a form of exercise or movement that brings you closer to ways in which you can love on yourself and your body.

No one can decide this for you! I personally LOVE to lift weights. I mean LOVE IT! Why? Because it calms my crazy little ADHD self right down. To me, the gym is like a sanctuary. Also, over all the years of being a self-professed "gym rat," I know there is NOTHING that sculpts a hot physique like weight training. And now at the age of 50, I have seen the results over and over again with both clients and friends who adopt the Living Sexy Fit Lifestyle.

What about you? What do you really enjoy to do? You've got to know what turns you on in the movement department, 'cause if you don't, the TV and a box of Girl Scout Cookies are going to be way more appealing! Ain't this the truth???

So, let's do a little investigating to get to the truth on what will *inspire you* to live all in with the super important exercise component of the Living Sexy Fit Plan. The bottom line is this: If you don't get to the "why" on what is in your way of living the LSF Lifestyle, no diet, trainer, or exercise plan is going to work. Notta' one!

You are the center of the Living Sexy Fit Plan, and if you are worried that this is going to be just one of those times when you start something and don't finish it, and then proceed to beat yourself up over another "failure," then it is time to dig a little deeper to what is in your "WHY". It's time to kiss your old self-defeating patterns goodbye once and for all! Ready?

Please answer the following questions:

1. What did you love to do as a little tyke, at your earliest memory?

2. How about at age 12?

3. At age 25?

4. Thinking back on your childhood, what did you love to do for physical activities? Did it take place inside or outside? With one other person, with a group, or solo?

5. Do you remember being a morning or night person? How about now, what are you?

6. What gave you joy as a child?

7. Where do you remember feeling the most safe and peaceful?

Great job on this! Any cool discoveries for you? Please fill them in here...

"All right, Kate, this is feeling a little like therapy... Really?... Why does my childhood have anything to do with why I hate to exercise and why I am overweight and out of shape??"

The reason why I ask these questions is that often it is an *inner voice* from our past, something that upended our confidence in our ability to shine brightly, that threw us off track. So what we need to do is remember – remember, so we can set ourselves free from old and outdated thoughts and feelings.

Once we set ourselves free from the untruths of the past, and reclaim our innate joy, we can now experience feeling powerful and celebratory in how we show up *today*. It's time to reclaim our rock-star status and live the lives of joy and freedom we deserve!

Now let's translate those positive emotional memories into creating an exercise and movement plan that you will be able to not only commit to but also enjoy. Finding the right exercise plan that fits into your lifestyle is key to getting and keeping your sexy self blazing.

Being Fit is About Living Your Joy From the Inside Out!

Please circle any exercises listed below that you would like to incorporate in your life, and start creating a plan to try them out and have these activities become a part of your regular routine. Circle away.

Here's a partial list of possible solo exercise modalities.

walking	treadmill
running	weight lifting
biking	yoga
roller skating	stretching
dancing in your kitchen	stair climbing

Here are some group exercise opportunities:

Zumba	running clubs
CrossFit	spinning
aerobics	racquet sports
line dancing	basketball
aerobics	soccer
slow flow yoga	other competitive team sports

Kate's Living Sexy Fit Truth:

Living Sexy Fit begins with self-love and acceptance at the deepest level. Trust in your inner sanctum or whatever space brings you to your deepest peace and knowing.

Where is that space for YOU? Where do you feel the deepest level of peace and joy? This feeling is the core of the Living Sexy Fit journey. Inner confidence and self-awareness are SEXY!

Sure you will have setbacks on your Living Sexy Fit journey. But view every setbacks and stumble as opportunities to learn and grow.

I was often criticized for my blind-faith optimism. However, I have come to realize that this "resiliency muscle," as I like to call it, has been the key to my success not only in my fitness journey, but in life.

Staying true to who you are is the magic bullet to living an amazing breakthrough life. Letting go of self-sabotaging habits and beliefs is not easy, but it is so worth it!

Be your AMAZING self. The world awaits!

Living Sexy Fit   by Kate McKay

CHAPTER 19

The Living Sexy Fit Buff Body Plan

THE FIVE COMPONENTS OF FITNESS

"Knowing is not enough: we must apply. Willing is not enough: we must do."
~Goethe

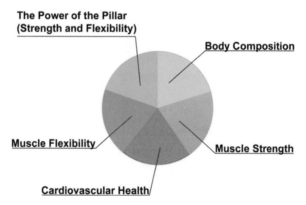

In order to achieve maximum bang for your buck with the Living Sexy Fit Buff Body Program, it is important for you to understand and embrace the five components of fitness. I have found that applying these five elements is crucial to achieving *optimal hotness*.

Being fit is defined by how well your body performs in each of these five categories:

1. The Power of the Pillar (Pillar Strength & Flexibility) –The pillar of the body is the foundation from which all movement stems. "Pillar is all the muscles that connect your hips, torso, and shoulders," *Mark Verstegen When these areas are poorly aligned, problems, can occur throughout all activities that you engage in.

   Think about it – when you twist an ankle, pull your back, or strain a shoulder, your whole movement pattern is affected. Injuries of the elbows and knees are often caused by breaks in movement patterns originating in the pillar. That it is why it is so crucial to stay fluid, strong, and flexible in the hip and shoulder areas.

   Action: Stretch your hips and shoulders throughout the day. Stand and move around every 20 minutes if you have a sedentary job. Reach your arms out and around, roll your neck, shake out your hips doing circles. Full dance boogie breakout is encouraged!

2. Muscle Flexibility. Muscle flexibility is defined as the ability of each and every joint, muscle, and tendon to move through its full range of motion. Exercises that promote flexibility include yoga, Pilates, stretch class, and exercise band work.

   As we age, we tend to stretch less, making us more prone to aches and pains, not to mention injury, falls, and strains. Please be the exception to this rule! Keep the body limber and flexible to maintain a youthful and flexible physique.

   Action: A healthy muscle is a strong and flexible one. Celebrate moving all of your joints through full range of motion. Smile and sigh as you stretch. Stiffness is a common sensation that needs to be worked through daily to completely unleash your sexy fit. Embrace your ability to move and groove!

3. Muscle Strength. Muscle strength describes how much force a muscle can exert. In general, the best way to increase your muscle strength is through strength training – my personal favorite. I view strength training as our own unique ability to play Michelangelo with these beautiful bodies we call our own. All bodies are different; they provide us with unique strategies and challenges to optimize our beautiful machines.

   This is the exciting and ever-evolving part of strength training that excites me so much. It has been the reason why I have remained so actively committed to this form of exercise over the last 30 years.

   Action: In order to optimize your strength, include strength training in your exercise program. Strength-train for a minimum of three times a week for 30 minutes a session to experience the amazing benefits.

   Anyway, given the simple fact that the more muscle you have the more you can eat, I say, heck, why would anyone *not* lift weights??

4. Cardiovascular Health. Cardiovascular health describes how well your heart and lungs work together to fuel your body with oxygen to your muscles and how well your muscles use it during sustained physical exertion. We will talk further about the different types of cardio activities in a later chapter, but know that getting the heart and lungs pumping is the best way to get you in that fat-burning zone.

   Action: Include daily cardiovascular exercise in your daily routine by "hooking" it to other activities. Carry the laundry upstairs in multiple steps, dance while making dinner, jog to the end of the street before you grab your mail from your mailbox. Include a combination of sustained vigor and bursts of heart-pumping exercise every day. Go for the cardio glow!

Living Sexy Fit   by Kate McKay

5. Body Composition. Your body composition serves as a barometer of your overall health and fitness. It takes into consideration your ratio of body fat to lean mass (muscles, bones, and organs) and can be an indicator of possible health risks. Your Living Sexy Fit goal is to have an optimal lean-tissue-to-body-fat ratio.

    Action: The LSF Buff Body Program includes both cardiovascular activity and strength training to melt away your body fat and increase muscle mass for greater calorie burn. Having a leaner machine is a great indicator of overall fitness and health, and plus, you just feel better all around.

    There are numerous ways to test your lean muscle/body fat ration. I personally use the Omron Fat Loss Handheld Monitor on myself and my clients. It's easy to use and relatively inexpensive.

With the Living Sexy Fit Clean Eats Diet and Buff Body Exercise Plan, your hotness factor will be sizzling! Please re-read the five components again now, and be sure to occasionally review them as they are key indicators to measure your overall success.

Kate Fit Tip:

"Why should I eat so often?"

Despite what many of our mothers told us, research now shows that eating smaller, more frequent meals is the way to go. Eating more frequently elevates mood and concentration, helps retain muscle mass and, conversely, you lose more body fat. So please, snack away your five meals. This old adage no longer applies.

CHAPTER 20

The Living Sexy Fit Buff Body System

STRENGTH-TRAIN YOUR WAY TO HOTNESS AND HEALTH!
BENEFITS OF STRENGTH TRAINING

There are no ifs, ands, or buts about it: Strength training is an amazing way to shape your body. The health benefits of pumping weights have been shown over and over again in numerous studies.

Research proves that women who engage in a regular strength training program enjoy a long list of health benefits. Unfortunately, unless we continue to perform regular strength training exercises, we lose more than ½ pound of muscle every year of life after age 25. Yikes!

What does that tell us about our weight gain as so many of us age? Yup, we gain dreaded fat, and at the same time we lose precious muscle!

EEK! *Now* do you see why I am so passionate about the importance of strength training??

A comprehensive strength training program that addresses all major muscle groups is a great way to prevent injury and degenerative diseases. And nothing makes you feel more sexy than being fit!

Below, I have listed five of the many reasons why you should take strength training more seriously and why now is the time to hop on the iron-pumping bandwagon:

1. *Muscle fights obesity.* The more muscle you have, the more calories you burn, even when you are sleeping! Each pound of muscle actually burns an extra 35 to 50 calories a day. A pound of fat burns only 2 calories a day. Yucko! Bring on the muscle!
2. *Strength training increases overall strength and energy for daily activities.* Weight training increases spinal bone density in as little as six months of training, thereby preventing osteoporosis.
3. *Strength training reduces risk of diabetes and heart disease.* Studies show that strength training increases glucose/blood sugar utilization by approximately 25% in four months. Also, stronger muscles lead to a stronger heart and decrease the risk of heart attack and heart disease.
4. *Strength training fights back pain and arthritis.* Lifting weights reduces chronic pain. It increases muscle strength, making us more able to stand and move in correct posture and alignment, and makes us more readily able to perform daily activities pain-free.
5. *Strength training reduces depression and anxiety.* A Harvard study found that 10 weeks of strength training reduced clinical depression symptoms. You just feel more confident and capable after a workout, and that translates into a happier state of being.

Certainly the health benefits are well documented. From my own personal experience, nothing in my life has made me feel more centered and powerful than the experience of a great workout.

Do I personally always love exercise session? Of course not. But do I like the way it makes me look and feel? Heck, yeah. It is the main reason why I am so passionate about inspiring others to be fit: So that they too can experience the amazing feelings of being in complete flow with their bodies and of being both strong and powerful.

Being strong is way sexier than being skinny!

Be ready to see your body change in ways that will surprise you. Notice how your inner confidence shifts. Observe how your stress level decreases. Be ready for your sex drive to increase. Trust me! These things really do happen! I hear it all the time from my happy clients.

Strength Training 101
The Living Sexy Fit Way!

For maximum results, and to prevent injury, please follow these guidelines as you work through your strength training program:

1. *Warm Up.* "Cold muscles" are more susceptible to injury. Start your workout session with light aerobic activity, such as a few minutes on the treadmill or light calisthenics like jumping jacks, arm circles, toe touches, or *dynamic stretches* that loosen the muscles.

2. *Focus on Form.* Correct form is crucial to prevent injury and to attain maximum gains when lifting weights. It is important to perform each exercise through a full range of motion, emphasizing the "squeeze" in the muscle at maximum contraction. Don't rush! Working through the whole range of motion reaps the greatest benefits.

3. *Use Enough Resistance.* Nothing drives me crazier than seeing someone lift a 5-lb. weight when they can manage 2 to 3 times that weight! Don't make me come find you, lol! Your goal in your strength training program is to work the targeted muscle to fatigue. Lift the appropriate amount of weight to challenge your body for optimal hotness. I know you want the gains. It is time for you to go after them.

4. *Listen to your Body.* Breathe, stretch between sets, tune in to how your body is feeling. Pay attention to pinches or strains. Notice where you feel tight and stiff, and use your weight training time to work through these tight areas. Stay tuned in to your form for maximum benefit. And if something hurts or pulls, please stop that exercise and move onto another. Respect what your body tells you, but always continue to challenge your body past its previous plateau.

5. *Push through Fear and Resistance.* This is probably the stickiest point for newbies as they start to lift weights. The key is this: the body will follow what the mind sets out to do. Believe that you can make the gains you desire, and your body will follow suit. Sometimes you reach a point where your mind will try to psyche you out and you will doubt your ability to move heavier weights. It is important to visualize yourself going through the exercise, breathe and dig in. You will be in awe of how quickly they improve when you fully commit to the best version of you! Trust and believe!

Important Living Sexy Fit Tip:

The Difference between Dynamic and Static Stretching:

Dynamic Stretching: This type of stretching is performed at the beginning of your workout to get the body ready to move and groove. Dynamic stretches closely mimic movements made during exercise. They are shorter in duration than static stretches, and are done while the body is in motion.

Static Stretching: Static stretching is low-force, long-duration stretching that holds the desired muscles at their greatest possible extension for 15 to 30 seconds. Static stretches are used to improve flexibility and cool your body down after you exercise, and are therefore done when the body is standing still.

Strength Training Guidelines
(Boring, but Important!)

When performing your strength training workout, please consider the following guidelines:

1. *Exercise Selection:* Select at least one exercise for each major muscle group to ensure that your muscle development is balanced. Please consult the exercises in Chapter 23.

2. *Exercise Sequence:* Vary your exercise sequencing when performing your workout.

   Oftentimes, we work from larger to smaller muscle groups starting with the larger muscle groups (chest, back, quadriceps, hamstrings, glutes) and work the smaller muscle groups after (biceps/triceps, calves); or we can switch things up by working upper and lower body in different work outs on different days.

   Please note in the Living Sexy Fit Buff Body Exercise Plan in the back of the book how the progression varies but always starts with the larger muscle groups; generally it's the best weight training progression.

3. *Exercise Sets and Repetitions:* A set is defined as a number of "reps" (repetitions) performed of a given exercise. In the Living Sexy Fit plan,

you will start by performing each series of exercises for one or two sets. Performing three sets of each exercise is for the more advanced Buff Body Babe. Go at your own pace and work up gradually in the number of sets you perform to avoid injury and risk overtraining.

4. *Exercise Progression:* The key to experiencing strength gains is applying "progressive resistance" to your exercise program. Once a muscle adapts to a certain amount of resistance, you will need to switch things up to keep the body guessing. For example, an ideal rep range in a set is lifting the weight between 8 and 12 times. When you can perform 12 reps with relative ease, it is time to increase the weight that you are lifting by about 5%. To make the gains, keep your body in "shock and awe." Just an in our intimate relationships, it is important to keep things fresh by switching things up. This same principle applies to your gym time as it does to the bedroom.

Remember: Strong Is Sexy!

Strength Training Chapter Summary

1. Warm up! Be kind to your body by preparing it for action. You want to heat up those muscles so that you reduce the chance of injury. Please don't miss this important step.

2. Perform dynamic stretches at the beginning of your workout to get your body ready to move into greater action.

3. Work through the full range of motion of the muscle, never jerking the weight.

4. Make the last set your most challenging set. Don't be surprised by quivering and twitching muscles. That means they are waking up and growing! This is good!

5. Listen to your body, breathe through your exercise program, and enjoy your time in the gym. You will never regret a workout, so commit to the process and go at it with passionate conviction! You are worth it!

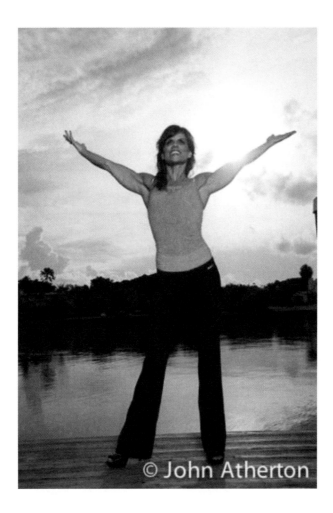

CHAPTER 21

The Living Sexy Fit Buff Body Cardio System

CARDIOVASCULAR EXERCISE – GO FOR THE GLOW!

When starting <u>any</u> exercise program, it is recommended that you make an appointment with your doctor to get the go-ahead on moving forward on your lifestyle changes and fitness goals.

Cardiovascular health is a crucial element of the Living Sexy Fit Program. We gotta' get the heart pumping to fully embrace our hotness factor!

The benefits of performing cardiovascular exercise include these:

- decreased blood pressure
- improved glucose tolerance
- reduced anxiety
- decreased risk of cardiovascular disease and diabetes

- increased vitality and elevated mood
- increased sex drive

As you can see, being in good cardiovascular health is the foundation of your fitness program and a crucial element in your overall health and your ability to enjoy your life, from playing with your kids to the ease at which you tackle your everyday tasks to even having a more fulfilling sex life!

Yahoo!

The Components of a Cardiovascular Work-Out

When we talk about taking cardiovascular exercise, we are referring to how well our heart, lungs, and circulatory system work together for optimal health and glow.

There are four elements that make up a rocking cardio plan, including:

1. mode
2. frequency
3. duration
4. intensity

of our cardiovascular plan.

Let's start from the top.

Mode: When we talk of our mode in our cardio program, we are talking about what cardio we will perform based on our interest, availability of time, and availability of equipment, and on our fitness goals. It is necessary that we figure out what will personally work for us so we can ensure that we will stay committed to the Living Sexy

Fit Plan. Don't choose the elliptical if you absolutely hate it! Being able to adhere to your mode of exercise and being clear on what you like and don't like is key.

Frequency: Frequency is deciding how many cardio sessions you are going to do each week. The American College of Sports Medicine recommends that we perform three to five days a week for most aerobic activities. In the Living Sexy Fit program, we focus on getting back to basics, incorporating more movement each and every day, and incorporating a more structured cardio session into our exercise regimen.

My questions to you when we talk about frequency are, "Are you committed to being Sexy Fit? To finally lose the extra fat that weighs you down? To embracing a more joy-filled lifestyle and feeling sexier and more vibrant?" If you are saying "yes, yes!" to these challenges, then it is time for you to commit to doing your cardio with more frequency so to attain the body you desire. You are worth it.

Duration: Duration refers to the number of minutes you perform your cardiovascular exercise in one session. Beginners, those who are just introducing or reintroducing more cardio and movement in their lives, should begin with 10- to 15-minute sessions. Intermediate fitness babes should be working up to the 40- to 60-minute zone, for maximum fat burn. Listen to your body! Reduce the length of cardio you are performing if suddenly feel dizzy or experience lightheadedness.

Intensity: Intensity measures the speed or the workload of the exercise you are performing. The American College of Sports Medicine recommends an intensity range of 55% to 90% of maximum heart rate. The wide variable in this range highlights the importance of your consulting with your physician for a full checkup. I recommend also meeting with a fitness professional, who can perform a fitness assessment on you to determine a recommended

Living Sexy Fit   by Kate McKay

level of exertion during your cardiovascular exercise and strength training program.

These professionals will be able to take into consideration your body composition, your age, your overall health, and any health risks and/or injuries to create an ideal cardio target exertion goal.

Keeping your focus on the intensity of your exercise means staying intentional to your goals *even* and *especially* when you don't feel like it. And if this isn't your first round on the fitness and health rodeo, those times do come!

Be prepared by staying clear in your goals and keeping up the intensity of your commitment to maximize your gains! Woo hoo!

Monitoring Exercise Intensity the Living Sexy Fit Way!

As a fitness professional, I most often monitor my clients' levels of exertion and how hard to push them based on what we in the industry call the **"talk test."** By paying attention to how my clients are breathing and how quickly they recover, I can pace their workouts accordingly. You can do the same thing for yourself.

Paying attention to your breathing is a great way for you to tune in to your own workouts. More on this when we talk about Borg's Rate of Exertion later in this chapter.

Another method of measuring exertion is the **Training Heart Rate Method.** This is calculated by subtracting your age from 220. Your training heart rate (THR) is your maximum measured heart rate multiplied by 60% to 90%.

For example: A 40-year-old woman for whom an intensity of 70% maximum heart rate is desired:

$$220 - 40 \text{ (age)} = 180 \text{ (predicted maximum heart rate)}$$
$$\times \, 70\% \text{ or } 0.70$$
$$= 126 \text{ (targeted exercise heart rate)}$$

So as she is performing her cardio, 126 beats per minute would be her targeted rate for maximum benefit at 70% of maximum intensity. You can calculate your own THR by using the above formula.

Another way of measuring your own exertion is with **Borg's Rating of Perceived Exertion (RPE)**, my personal favorite and the method I mention to my clients most frequently.

Borg Rating of Perceived Exertion (RPE)
The Living Sexy Fit Way!

Level 1: I am watching TV, eating Cheetos.
Level 2: I am comfortable and could maintain this pace all day.
Level 3: I am still comfortable, but I am breathing a bit harder.
Level 4: I am sweating at little, but I feel good and can carry on a conversation effortlessly.
Level 5: I am just above comfortable, sweating more, and can still talk with relative ease.
Level 6: I can still talk, but I am slightly breathless.
Level 7: I can still talk, but I don't really want to. I am sweating.
Level 8: I can grunt in response to your questions and can keep this pace for only a short time.
Level 9: I think I am dying. Gasp!
Level 10: What happened? Overexertion!

For maximum benefit in your cardio and exercise routine,
play in levels 5 to 8.

It is so important as you embrace your fitness journey that you take responsibility for your health and monitor your efforts to be sure you are not under-challenging yourself as much as you are not over-challenging yourself.

Being overzealous certainly is dangerous when exercising, because it does increase your chance of injury; however, under-challenging yourself is also an issue with people just starting exercise programs.

This happens for a variety of reasons:

- fear of pain
- feeling self-conscious
- dislike of sweating
- fear of wrecking our hair-do (truth!)
- fear of success
- even fear of extreme hurt or death

Seriously, these fears and emotions are real! My job as a coach and fitness trainer is so much more than helping people attain buff body status. Ask any trainer!

These fears and emotional challenges that hinder our progress are exactly why I am so passionate about doing the work that I do, by helping people just like you to embrace their fears, excavate their motivational mojo, and live the life of their dreams!

People just like YOU, who are READY to LIVE SEXY FIT!

To get fit and live your breakthrough life, you have to stay uncomfortable! Stay focused on your ultimate goals and keep moving!

Variety is the Spice of Life!
Different Aerobic Training Methods the Living Sexy Fit Way

Let's talk about three different aerobic training methods that you can use to get your game on and get your buff body moving and grooving. They are continuous training, interval training, and circuit training.

Continuous Aerobic Training is when your intensity remains between 50% and 85% of functional capacity (5 to 8 on Borg's scale). Shoot for 20 to 60 minutes as the ideal for maximum fitness improvement and body fat reduction. Remember that the intensity needs to be enough to get you in that fat-burning zone, so stay tuned in to your breathing and play in the higher end of your exertion scale for more effective gains.

Interval Training or HIIT TRAINING (high-intensity interval training) combines higher and lower levels of intensity throughout a cardio session. An example of this style of training is a spinning class or varied intervals on the treadmill, elliptical, bike, or track.

HIIT training has been shown to be very effective at increasing your metabolic rate; however, because of the greater intensity, it is important that you receive clearance from your doctor before you take on this style of conditioning.

Perform HIIT initially for a 10-minute session, then move to a minimum of 20 minutes and a maximum of 40 minutes to get your heart pumping and your metabolic rate churning.

Circuit Training is a great method of exercise that produces quicker gains by moving through a series of exercises with relatively brief rest periods between each station.

The cool thing about circuit training is that you can use strength training and cardio stations in combination, or a variety of cardiovascular exercises, in a single session to mix things up and keep the body guessing for maximum benefit and fitness gains.

Example of a Cardio/Strength Sequence:

Warmup on treadmill: 5 minutes
Body-weight squats: 1 minute (AMAP – as many as possible)
Treadmill: 5 minutes
Pushups on bench: 1 minute (AMAP)
Treadmill: 5 minutes
Ab crunches: 1 minute (AMAP)
Complete!

You can repeat this cycle two to three times. Feel free to change up the cardio modality. Choose exercises from Chapter 23 in the Living Sexy Fit book.

Example of Cardio Circuit Only:

Treadmill: 5 minutes
Stationary bike: 5 minutes
Elliptical: 5 minutes
Complete!

For an intermediate workout, repeat this cycle two to three times for maximum fat-burning and metabolism-boosting gain!

As you can see, there are many ways to shake things up when you embrace the Living Sexy Fit Buff Body Lifestyle. As with anything in life, it is important to switch things up to keep your body and mind guessing. To me, this is way more fun than a Sudoku puzzle!

Not only does change-up prevent boredom to set in, but it is also crucially important in my making the quickest gains to LIVING SEXY FIT!

Variety Is the Spice of Life! Live It!

Kate Gets Real!

Those who know me know that cardio is not my favorite! It's the truth!!! But in order to be in optimal health, and because heart disease runs in my family, I have come to embrace cardiovascular exercise.

I have found ways that work for me so I can perform this exercise mode with greater ease and less angst. What I have chosen to do is add more cardio bursts throughout my day: a brisk 15-minute walk with my pup, an extra set of stairs as I bring laundry up and down, a sprint to the mailbox, a longer treadmill warm-up before my weight training session. This works for me.

What will work for you? Investigate what you like to do or can tolerate (lol) and make a plan to get your body in action.

Cardio Health = Increased Stamina = Less Fatigue = Less Injury = More Fun!

If I Can Do It, You Can Do It, Too!

Exercise Tips to Remember:

- *Stop exercising immediately when you experience chest discomfort, numbing of limbs, light-headedness, or dizziness.*
- *Reduce exercise intensity in very hot or humid conditions.*
- *Avoid exercise with pain in a joint that only gets worse as you exercise.*

- *If you are under the care of a doctor for a chronic medical condition, obtain clearance from the doctor before proceeding with this or any exercise program.*

Hottie Hazard! "I don't have time to warm up! I am just going to go all out in this exercise class or weight training program!"

Please don't!!! It is crucial that you gradually increase your heart rate, your blood pressure, your oxygen consumption, and the elasticity of your muscles and joints to prevent injury and health risks. Be kind to your body! Warm it up with care!

CHAPTER 22

Living Sexy Fit Motivational Mojo and Exercise – *It's Not About Finding Time; It's About Making Time!*

TIPS TO MAKING THE TIME TO WORK OUT:

1. *Pack your workout bag the night before.* Truth: I have been known to wear my workout clothes to bed. Also, if I know I won't be hitting the gym until the end of the day, I will wear one piece of clothing that is fitness-related under my clothes, even if it is just my sports bra, to remind myself of my commitment to my fit time.

2. *Pack your pre-workout meal/snack the night before*, so you can grab it and go in the morning. Have you ever said to yourself, "I will just stop at home and grab something to eat," and found yourself in your pajamas in front of the TV covered in Doritos dust three hours later? Be prepared and avoid this serious Hottie Hazard.

3. *Plan on it!* Set your workout schedule for the month and stick to it. Make a commitment to your best and highest Sexy Fit self. For real, the weight-loss journey is not an easy one; if it were, we would all be skinny. Rid yourself of roadblocks that prevent you from getting to the gym by making this date with yourself non-negotiable.

4. *Find an accountability pal.* This is so crucial to your success! Share your LIVING SEXY FIT Commitment Contract with a trusted coach or friend and be sure to tell WHY you want to achieve these goals. Remember: The WHY is the firewood in your furnace of attaining your dreams.

5. *Get more done in less time with HIIT training.* The trend is toward shorter and more intense exercise sessions for a quicker fat burn and metabolism boost. The whole idea to HIIT training is to keep the body's fat-consuming furnace on high and put demands on the body to keep it guessing what is next. You can do this in a couple of different ways:

   a. Perform cardio in bursts at high intensity for, say, 30 seconds, then slow down until your heart rate drops back to a light jog rate, then boost it up for 30 to 50 seconds, repeating this for 25 to 30 minutes four to five times a week.

   b. Combine the cardio component with weights to really jack up your cardio and muscle-building machine. For example, perform 1 minute of cardio equipment followed by 20 squats, then go back to the cardio for 1 to 2 minutes at a high-intensity pace, then do a barbell chest press and then go back to cardio component, repeating this process for 20 to 30 minutes. Mix it up for maximum fat-burning, muscle-building fun!

CHAPTER 23

The Living Sexy Fit Exercise Program

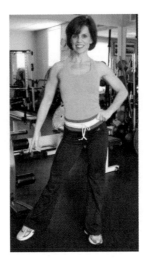

Perfect Posture:

The proper stance for optimal movement! Shoulder blades are back and down. The tummy is drawn up and in, activating the core muscles. Imagine a straight line from the ears to the shoulders, from the shoulders to the hips, from the hips to the knees, and from the knees to the ankles. Energy is rising out the top of your head!

Practice in front of the mirror first with your eyes open, and then try it with your eyes closed. Incorporate this long and lean vision all day long.

Athletic Stance:

The proper form for all sport and lifestyle movement. Start with holding perfect posture. Keep your legs slightly bent, with your bootie sitting slightly back and down. The weight is toward the front of the feet. Your core is engaged.

You are ready to roll!

EXERCISE SERIES

Suitcase Squats

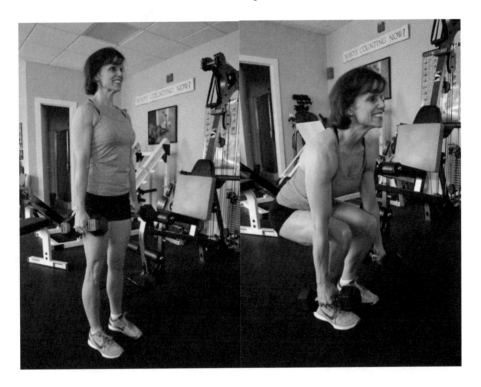

1. Holding a dumbbell in each hand, stand in perfect posture, with your shoulder blades down and back, chest lifted, and core engaged.

2. Slowly bring the weights down toward the floor, keeping the chest lifted and shifting the weight back on your heels, your glutes sticking out and back.

3. As you come up, keep the chest lifted and your weight on the heels. At the top, give the glutes a good squeeze. Repeat.

Living Sexy Fit   by Kate McKay

Sumo Plie Squats

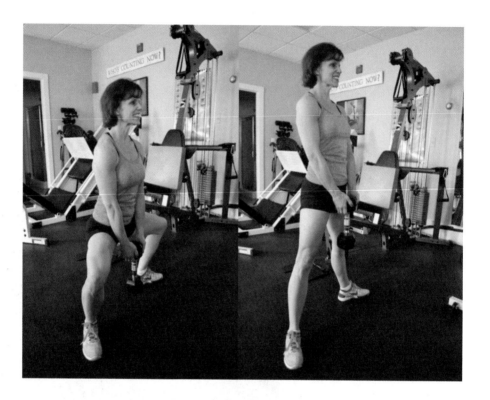

Step out into a wide stance with your feet turned out, parallel to your knees. Rotate out only as far as you are comfortable.

1. While holding a dumbbell with two hands, slowly lower down into a plié, keeping the weight distribution toward your heels. Do not let your knees rotate in.

2. When you are coming back up, activate the glutes, imagining energy coming out the top of your head. Give the glutes a squeeze at the top. Repeat.

Living Sexy Fit   by Kate McKay

Lunges (with dumbbells)

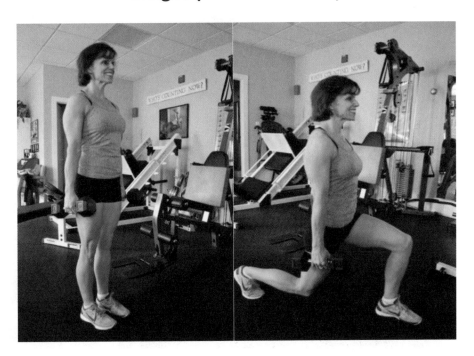

1. Standing in perfect posture, with your shoulders back and down, dumbbells by your side, step out with the left foot with a wide but comfortable step.

2. While you're in this posture, being sure your body weight is on the heel of the front foot, bend the back knee, lowering your body down until you feel a stretch in the front hamstring. Be sure the front knee does not pass the foot.

3. Lift your body up and back to the start position, pushing up and away and back to standing position, feet together. Repeat, leading with the other leg.

Dead Lift (Hamstring and Glutes)

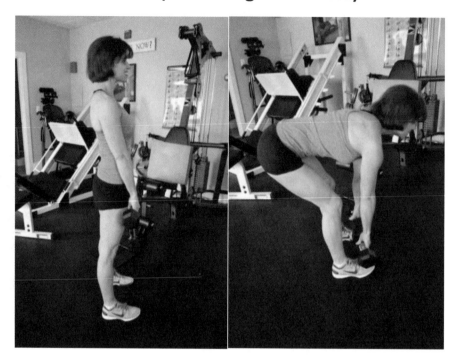

1. Start with the dumbbells facing your thighs, your knees slightly bent, your chest lifted, and your core engaged.

2. As you breathe in, slowly lower the weights toward the floor, keeping the weights close to the body and keeping your back straight. You should feel a stretch in the back of the legs.

3. Once you have reached as low as you can go, feeling a nice stretch in the hamstrings, blow out as you squeeze your glutes and bring the weights up alongside your legs. Be sure the weight is on the heels.

> **TIP:**
> Keep the weight on the heels of the feet.

Calf Raises

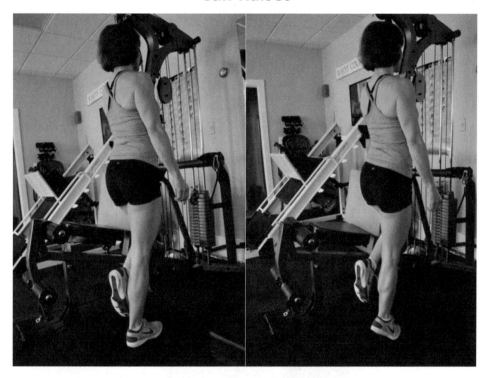

1. Stand on one leg. Hold onto a steady object for balance.

2. Slowly lift up onto your toe to full extension, blowing out as you rise. Then slowly lower yourself with a controlled movement. Repeat.

Variation: You can also try this holding a dumbbell in your free hand.

Pushups (Chest, Triceps)

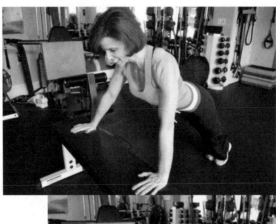

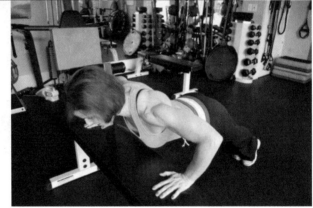

1. Start by placing your hands slightly wider apart than your shoulders on a bench, counter, or chair. Walk your feet out so that you are in a plank position as shown in position 1 above.

2. With your core activated and with energy coming out of your head, slowly lower your chest to the bench.

3. Slowly press with the palms of the hands and blow out as you push your chest away from the bench. Repeat.

Dumbbell Press (Chest)

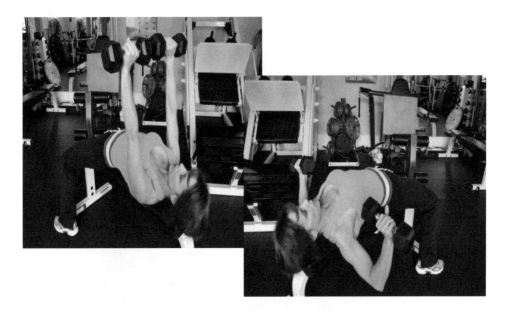

1. Lie on a bench with the dumbbells by your chest, creating a V with each arm, feeling a nice stretch through the shoulders and chest.

2. While breathing out, push the dumbbells up until your arms are essentially extended above your chest (level with your nipples). Slowly lower the weights down as you breathe in.

> **TIP:**
> Don't over-grip the dumbbells. Keep your hips planted on bench.

> **TIP:**
> Keep the chest lifted and slightly arch your back.

Dumbbell Flyes (Chest)

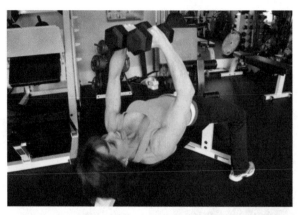

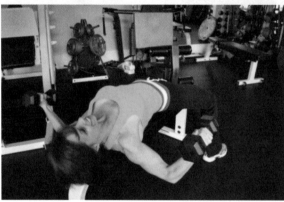

1. Lying flat on the bench, hold the dumbbells above your chest so they are touching each other and your arms are extended but bent, as if you are hugging a barrel.

2. Inhale as you lower the weights to either side; your arms will remain fixed in their barrel-hugging angle, and the weights will arc outward as they come down. Be careful not to bring the dumbbells too low. Now, breathing out, return to the start position.

Bent-Over Dumbbell Rows

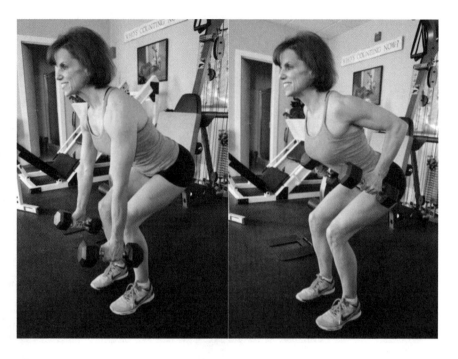

1. While standing in your athletic stance, bend at the hips with the dumbbells in front of you, facing each other.

2. As you breathe in, bring the dumbbells up and back along your body, elbows lifting, chest lifted.

> **TIP**:
> Keep your face and chest open and up, and your core activated.

Dumbbell Military Press (Shoulders)

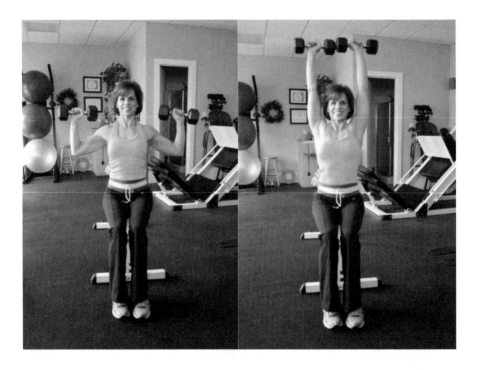

1. To begin, lift the dumbbell over *and* above your shoulders with the elbows bent, again forming V's with your arms.

2. As you blow out, lift the weights in a semicircle over your head with a smooth movement. Lower the weight to the start position in a controlled pace with your chest lifted.

> **TIP**:
> Keep your chest lifted. Be careful not to over-grip the weights.

Lateral Raises (Shoulders)

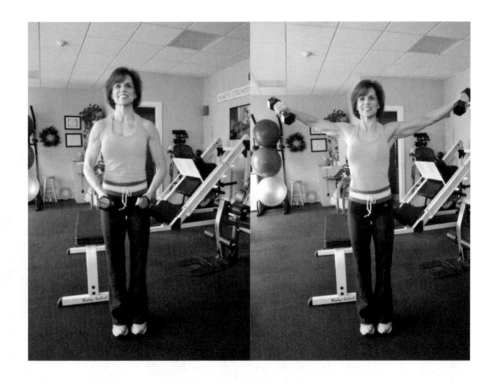

1. Hold the dumbbells at your hips facing in, your elbows and knees slightly bent. Bend slightly forward at the waist. You are in the athletic stance.

2. As you breathe out, raise the weights out to the side, imagining that you are holding two pitchers in each hand. As you raise the weight, pretend that you are pouring something out of the pitchers at the top phase of the repetition. Breathe in as you lower the weights.

> **TIP:**
> Keep your knees slightly bent through this exercise, and your core engaged.

Rear Bent Raises (Shoulders)

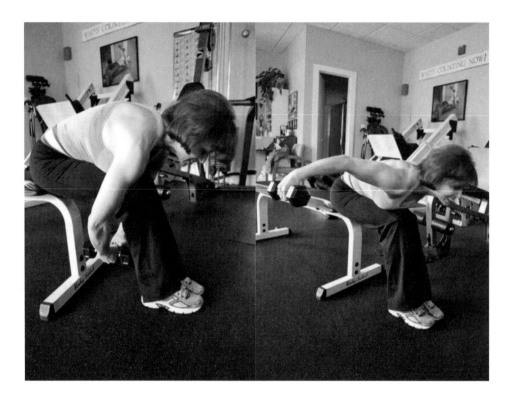

1. Sit on the bench, holding the dumbbells facing each other underneath your legs, keeping your elbows slightly bent.

2. Pressing your chest forward into your knees, lift the weights up and out, keeping the elbows slightly bent, blowing out on exertion.

> **TIP:**
> Use the same pitcher-pouring technique you do on the lateral raises.

Triceps Dumbbell Kick Backs

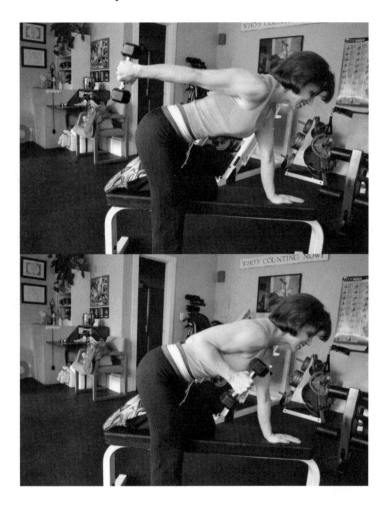

1. Start with one knee and the corresponding palm on the bench.

2. With a dumbbell in the opposite hand and the corresponding elbow pressed into your side, extend your arm straight back and squeeze the muscle in the back of your arm. Repeat.

Keep your core activated and your back straight throughout the exercise.

Bench Dips (Triceps)

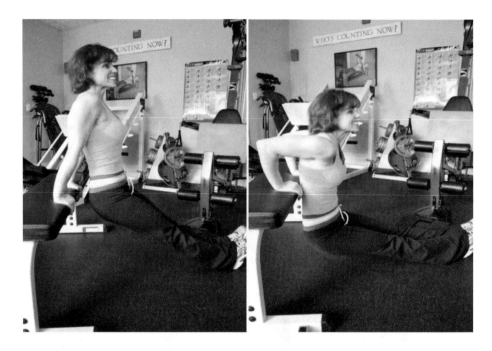

1. Start out sitting on the edge of the bench with your fingers facing your body. Lift your bootie off the bench as you walk your feet out a comfortable distance.

2. As you breathe in, lower your body along the bench, keeping your elbows in and back.

3. Once you have reached your full depth, blow out as you press up, straightening your arms.

> **TIP:**
> Remember to keep your body close to the bench as you
> do this exercise.

Dumbbell Curls (Biceps)

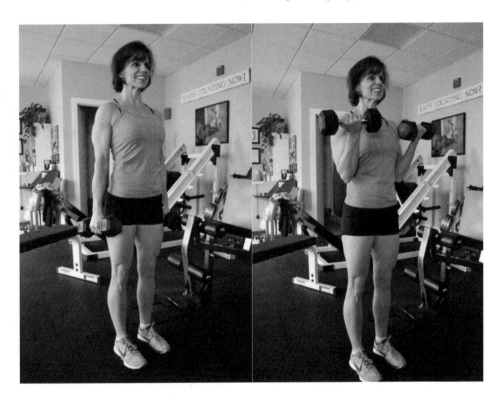

1. Hold the dumbbells by your side, weights along your body.

2. As you blow out, raise the weights up toward your shoulders, being aware of the contraction in the biceps.

3. Blow out as you lower the weights in a controlled and smooth motion.

TIP:
Be careful not to over-grip weights.

Living Sexy Fit   by Kate McKay

Six-Pack Abs Trio Set

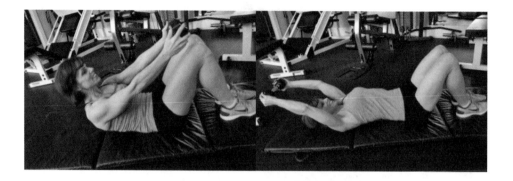

1. Start this exercise lying flat on your back and holding a light dumbbell overhead. As you blow out, lift your body slightly up off the mat. Imagine that your core is being scooped out like a scoop of gelato. Pause for two counts at the top of the exercise.

2. Lower the weight slowly back and away, with a slight bend in the elbow.

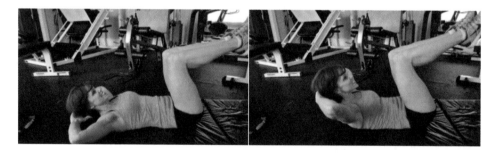

1. With your fingers gently resting on the back of your head and your elbows pressing out, slowly lift the chest up and out until you feel the core activating, particularly on the upper part of the abdomen, just below the ribs.

2. Keeping the elbows pressed back, lower your body to the mat, keeping the core activated throughout the up-and-down movement.

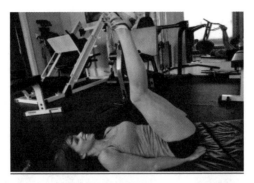

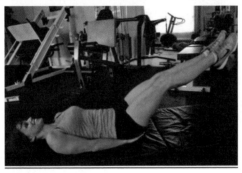

1. Lying flat on your back, rest your hands under your glutes, palms facing down, with your legs up and slightly bent.

2. Slowly lower the legs down toward the floor, contracting the lower abs. Lower your legs only as low as is comfortable, being cautious that you put no stress on the lower back.

3. Breathe in as you bring your legs back up to position 1. Repeat.

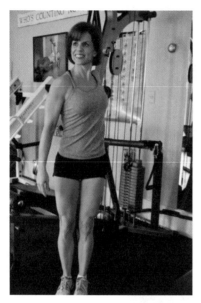

Chest Stretch

With the core activated and one shoulder blade back and down, grip a post with your hand and stretch away, feeling a great stretch in the shoulder and chest. Repeat with your other arm.

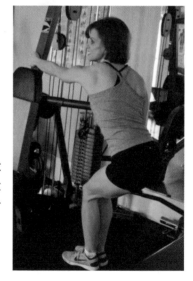

Lat Stretch

With the core active, grasp a pole and, with soft knees, lean your body away, feeling a great stretch through the upper back and rear shoulder.

Shoulder Stretch

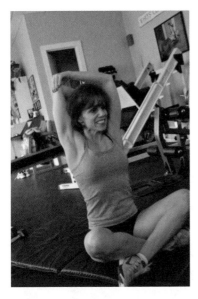

Either sitting or standing, grasp the opposing elbow with the opposite hand and pull the elbow back, bending slightly at the waist to intensify the stretch. Repeat on the other side.

Side Stretch

Breathe in deeply as you reach one arm up and over your head, feeling a stretch from the hip all the way through the armpit and blow out as you lean fully into the stretch. Repeat on the other side.

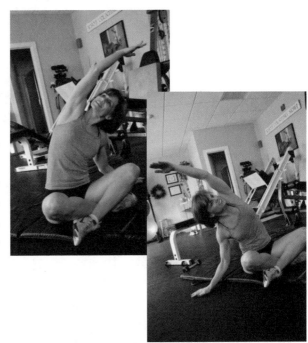

Hip Stretch 1

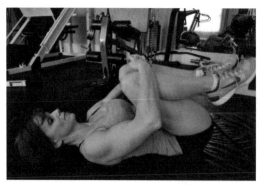

Lying flat on your back, gently bring your hips into your chest and hold for a count of 10. With each breath in and out, feel the hips release a little more. Rock gently back and forth, come to center, and then release the knees to the floor. Feel the weight of your body resting into the mat.

Hip Stretch 2

Lying on your back, rest one ankle on the opposing knee. Grasp behind the thigh and, blowing in and out, pull the leg toward the chest. You should feel the stretch in the hip and outer thigh of the crossed leg.

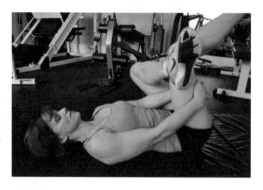

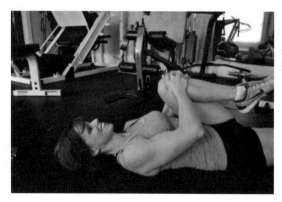

Hip Stretch 3

Lying on your back, gently bring one knee to the chest, imagining you are creating more space in that hip joint. Hold for 10 seconds. Rock slightly to the left and right. Release and rotate to the other side.

Hip Stretch 4

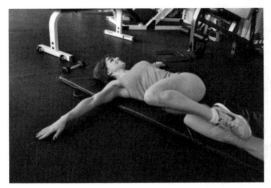

Lying flat on your back, bring one knee up and then gently drop the knee across the body, keeping the shoulder blades pressing into the mat. Focus on your breath, and feel the waist and hip open and release. Bring the leg back to center, lower the leg, and perform the stretch on the other side.

Hip Stretch 5

Sit with one leg straight out behind you and one leg bent in front, using your hands to monitor the intensity of the hip stretch. Breathe in and out, allowing the hip to release deeper with each breath. Repeat with the leg positions reversed.

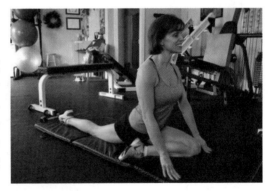

Hip Stretch 6a

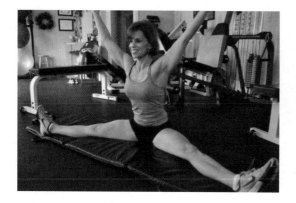

Hip Stretch 6b

1. Start with the legs a comfortable width apart in a sitting position. You can also perform this stretch with your back against a wall for extra support. Be sure that your feet are rotated slightly out and in line with your knees.

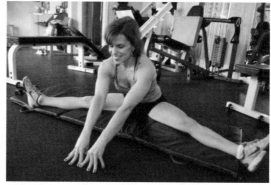

2. Breathing in, lift your arms up overhead and activate the core. Slowly bring your arms in front of you toward the floor, resting your fingertips for support. Breathe in and out as you feel the release in the hips. Move the fingers a little to the left and right to expand on the stretch.

3. Slowly walk your fingers in and raise your body up, then bring the legs together and shake them out. Repeat one to two times.

Inner Thigh Stretch 1

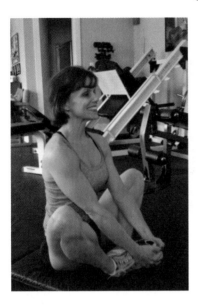

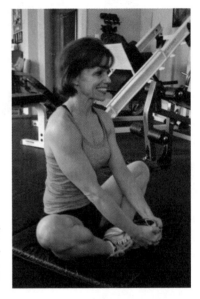

1. Sitting on the mat, bring the soles of your feet together and activate your core, keeping the shoulders back and down, chest lifted.

2. As you breathe out, lower the knees toward the mat. You can use the palms of the hands on the inside of the knees to increase the stretch. Repeat.

Inner Thigh Stretch 2

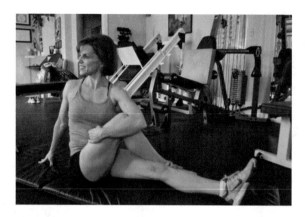

1. Sitting on the mat with your legs in front of you, bring one knee up and over the other knee.

2. Wrap the opposite arm around the knee and, with the free arm, reach around and rest your fingers on the mat.

3. Breathe in as you lift the chest and rotate the rib cage, feeling a great stretch in the hip and waist. Blow out all your breath when you reach the full stretch, hold, then release. Repeat on the opposite side, noticing how the stretch may feel different on each side. Breathe into any tight areas.

Hamstring Stretch 1-3

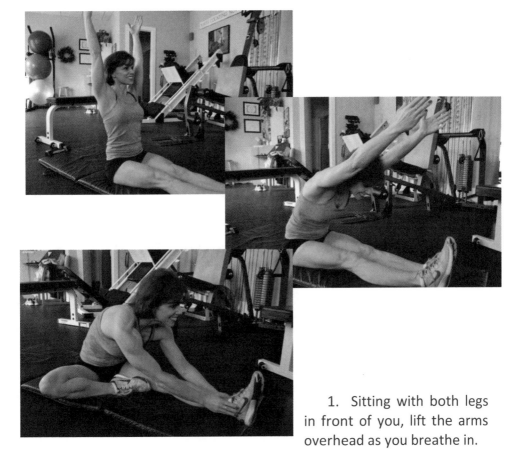

1. Sitting with both legs in front of you, lift the arms overhead as you breathe in.

2. As you release your breath, lean forward, imagining energy coming out of the top of your head. Do not slump into the stretch, and keep your core active.

Variation: bend one leg with the foot against the inside of the knee and hinge at your waist. Again, notice the difference, if any, in each hip. Breathe into any tight spots.

Living Sexy Fit   by Kate McKay

Check out my 28 Day Living Fabulously with Kate Program:

www.kate-mckay.com/products

Stay in action and remember, self-respect begins at the lips!

PART FIVE

Living Sexy Fit

Putting the Plan into Action

Living Sexy Fit   by Kate McKay

CHAPTER 24

Living the Sexy Fit Lifestyle –
Putting It All Together!

Are you ready to put it all together?

As we discussed throughout this book, being sexy fit takes a holistic approach by incorporating the mind, body, and soul of who you are at the deepest level and bringing all your good to the surface.

But first, in order to live a jacked up and yummy life, it's time for you to get real and get radical about what you will expect out of this amazing life you got going on. And frankly, it is due time you give your negative self-talk and nonsensical psycho-babble the boot! It serves you NOT and you know it.

By embracing the Living Sexy Fit lifestyle, be prepared for your life to change, possibly in all areas and facets. Expecting the shake-up will help you stay focused and committed to your highest and best kick-butt self, by being crystal clear on what you want, why you want it and having others who love you to support you on your journey.

I hear it all the time from clients, even friends: "Well Kate, you are just different, most people cannot do what you do, with the same passion, drive and desire." And my response is, "Are we talking about all these other people, or are we talking about you?" Why is it that when we feel like we cannot attain something we start talking about ourselves in the third person, the mysterious "other"?

So I ask you this: How bad do you want it? How bad do you want to feel hot and sexy? How bad do you want to have deep and meaningful relationships in your life? How bad to do you want to live with passion and financial abundance and a deep conviction that there is more than enough? How bad do you want to be free from self-sabotage and feelings of negative self-worth?

If you have read this far, then gosh darn it, you want it THAT BAD, and I want you to have all that you desire. And this is the core reason why I have written *Living Sexy Fit*: to inspire and challenge you to grow through emotional blocks and truly "see" yourself as the whole and healthy Hottie that you came here to be.

The truth is I will not let you settle for less than you deserve or desire. It is the success stories of my clients that drive me on a daily basis. To inspire you to have the courage and faith to live your life all out, with passion, confidence, and a sexy sizzle!

The first step is to set yourself free from negative self-talk and personal soul bashing. It is possible, I promise you, to be free of this self-defeating behavior. The biggest success will come to those who are finally ready to shift their self-perception, become aware of self-defeating language and behavior, and move into a place of positive self-worth and self-love. Positive mojo is a choice. Live it.

The second step of the Living Sexy Fit challenge is incorporating and embracing the clean eats diet program. By eating clean, you will become so in tune with your body, it will blow you away. Once you make the change to a healthy lifestyle, it is nearly impossible to turn back. You will see clearly that the best way to honor yourself is to honor the body you have been given to the highest level. You deserve it.

And lastly, by incorporating the Living Sexy Fit exercise plan, you will be able to create killer results and a chiseled physique by being your own Michelango. I believe there is no better way to have a shapely physique than to incorporate strength training.

Also by getting on a regular cardio plan, you will be able to see fat fall away and your health increase on all levels. And there is nothing sexier than the just-exercised glow!

Please do not cut yourself short. I want you to succeed, and I will do all that I can to ensure that this becomes a reality. I am here cheering you on every step of the way.

My Living Sexy Fit Tribe, I look forward to that day when we can meet each other and you can tell me all about your transformation. I look forward to us doing the happy dance together!

In celebration of your courage, strength, and willingness to go all in and lots, and lots of love,

Kate McKay

Your Land of Possibility...

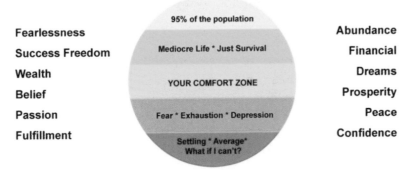

Fearlessness

Success Freedom

Wealth

Belief

Passion

Fulfillment

95% of the population

Mediocre Life * Just Survival

YOUR COMFORT ZONE

Fear * Exhaustion * Depression

Settling * Average*
What if I can't?

Abundance

Financial

Dreams

Prosperity

Peace

Confidence

The sky is the limit!

"It always seems impossible until it's done." —Nelson Mandela

Bringing it All Together – 10 Steps to the Living Sexy Fit Lifestyle!

1. Be disturbed!
2. Commit to your Living Sexy Fit transformation by releasing old patterns that no longer serve you.
3. Sign on the dotted line! Your Living Sexy Fit Commitment to YOU!
4. Purge your comfy fat clothes, hidden junk food, any food that leads you to binge.
5. Create your exercise sanctuary at home or join a gym where you are comfortable.
6. Create your weekly and monthly plans for success in exercise and meals.
7. Stay in Action!
8. Celebrate micro wins along the way!
9. Monitor your progress. Post your challenges and wins on Facebook.
10. Share your success with others! Over 67% of adults in our country are obese. Your successes will encourage and inspire others to live the Sexy Fit Lifestyle.

Vision Creation – Letting Loose Your Passion
Living in Alignment with Your True Vision

"Life is not measured by the number of breaths we take, but by the moments that take our breath away."
— Unknown

Putting yourself in the equation of your life takes courage. It also takes a plan.

You can float along the river, without a paddle, meandering through the waterways, thrown down rapids and waterfalls, and hitting dry land where you need to port, blistered and sunburned, cursing the world. *Or* you can get yourself an oar and a map, and create a life plan that "takes your breath away" with all that is juicy good.

Are you ready?

News Flash! Every **decision** you make leads to your **destiny**.

All the variables – divorce, job loss, states of feeling overwhelmed, 5-lb. holiday weight gain, stubbed toes, business stress, even unmanaged success – are just **conditions** of YOUR decisions you have made as to how to live your life.

And guess what that means?

Yup, YOU are in charge.

Victim consciousness, pity parties, poor me's – it's over. It's time to tune into your emotional barometer and create an action plan to get you sailing in the right direction.

So dig in, face the music, and do the work. ALL of it. Because when you fully realize that you are the commander in charge of your magnificent ship, your life will shift and lift in ways that you never thought were possible.

Tally HO!

1. List five things that take your breath away, fire you up, put you in a state of awe and wonder! Come on, I know it may be a long time, but you got this!

   1.
   2.
   3.
   4.
   5.

1. Circle the one you want more of, like, yesterday...

2. Now, create a plan as to how you are going to get it. Include one action for today, this week, this month, this year, to get you more of what you truly want and need to live a full and juicy life! You are worthy, so let's get busy!

Action Plan: I want

1. Today I will
    Action

    Milestone

    Action

2. This week I will
    Action

    Milestone

    Action

3. This month/year I will
    Action

    Milestone

    Action

Great job! It's that simple! If you want something, it is yours for the taking.

Congrats!

Now that we have played with visioning, let's set up some goals to get you on track to live all in!

Your Personal Living Sexy Fit Goals

My Living Sexy Fit Health & Wellness Goals I will put into action are:

1. _____
   _____
   _____
   _____

2. _____
   _____
   _____
   _____

3. _____
   _____
   _____
   _____

Remember: A goal is just a dream with a timeline!

1. Why is now the time for you to achieve these goals?
2. What has gotten in your way before?
3. How will you deal with obstacles, both old ones and new ones, that show up?
4. How will you celebrate your success?
5. Who will you celebrate with?
6. How will it feel to attain your fitness goals, once and for all?

Remember: Behind every successful person is a powerful support system of believers. As you move through your Living Sexy Fit transformation, think about who is currently on your team?

Who may need to go?

Who do you want to ask to join to support you?

The answers may surprise you!

Be honest!

Just because the people closest to you are not supporting you by jumping up and down with pom-poms does not mean that they do not love you. They did not sign up for this transformation, you did! Sure, they will benefit from this transformation in oodles of ways. But understand that no matter how you slice it, when someone changes, others around them are threatened, and that will certainly include those nearest and dearest to you.

Be prepared for negativity and outright hostility from others. Meet and greet these reactions with loving kindness. This is not always easy, but taking the high road is always the better choice.

I am not promoting putting up with rude behavior. Heck no! What I am saying is to realize that others negative baggage is not your issue, it is theirs. You can choose to create a healthy space around you so that you can stay focused on your goals. Surround yourself with people who support your dreams and buffer you from the less positive peeps. Lean on them when you need them. They will be happy to help!

Remember: Transformation = fear in people who love you = opportunity for you to be kind and gracious. Find positive peeps to keep you focused on your sexy fit goals.

On the flipside of this, as you transform and become more filled with self-love and self-acceptance, and gosh darn it, more HOT, relationships that you have been super-gluing to keep together often must be completely unglued to see if they are worth putting back together.

This may be the perfect opportunity for you to bring on a great coach or therapist to keep you clear and honest as you sort through the emotions that surface. They can also help you structure an action plan that keeps you committed and remind you of your "WHY" and the importance of staying on task to live your highest and best life.

Live By the Rule of Process Not Perfection

As you embark on your 28-Day Plan, live by the Rule of Process Not Perfection. Anticipate that there will be obstacles in your path. When you encounter them, embrace them as opportunities to learn to stay the course with your eating and training.

28-Day Living Sexy Fit Plan

Fit Plan for _____

Name

Address

Phone #

Email

Week 1: Date

Measurements: chest   hips   waist   left arm   left leg

Weight

Body Fat

Week 2: Date

Measurements: chest   hips   waist   left arm   left leg

Weight

Body Fat

Week 3: Date

Measurements: chest   hips   waist   left arm   left leg

Weight

Body Fat

Week 4: Date

Measurements: chest   hips   waist   left arm   left leg

Weight

Body Fat

Total Net Loss

Bravo!

My goal for the next 28 days is to

_____

_____

_____

_____

_____

This is important to me because

_____

_____

_____

_____

_____

The 28-Day Exercise Plan

Here are two sample training schedules for the 28-Day Plan, a beginner plan and an intermediate plan.

To get the most from it, make sure to increase the intensity of your efforts as your fitness level increases. You can have a Free Movement Day any day of the week – your choice. Just make sure you keep that time for yourself and use that day to restore, prep food, and get ready for an amazing Living Sexy Fit Lifestyle!

Remember: Fitness starts as an inside job. Realize you are worth the time, commitment, and love to let your wildest dreams come true!

Beginner Living Sexy Fit Buff Body Plan*

	Monday	Tuesday	Wednesday	Thursday	Friday	Saturday	Sunday
Week 1	Cardio 10 min	Weights: Upper Body	Cardio 15 min	Weights: Lower Body/Abs	Cardio 20 min	Weights: Upper Body	Free Movement Day
Week 2	Weights: Lower Body/Abs	Cardio 20 min	Weights: Upper Body	Cardio 30 min	Weights: Lower Body/Abs	Cardio 20 min	Free Movement Day
Week 3	Cardio 30 min	Weights: Upper Body	Cardio 30 min	Weights: Lower Body/Abs	Cardio 30 min	Weights: Upper Body	Free Movement Day
Week 4	Weights: Lower Body/Abs	Cardio 40 min	Weights: Upper Body	Cardio 20 min	Weights: Lower Body/Abs	Cardio 40 min	Free Movement Day

*Please refer to Appendix for Exercise Journals

Intermediate Living Sexy Fit Plan*

	Monday	Tuesday	Wednesday	Thursday	Friday	Saturday	Sunday
Week 1	Cardio 15 min Stretch	Weights: Upper Body Abs HIIT 6 min	Cardio 20 min Shoulders Stretch	Weights: Lower Body/Abs Abs HIIT 10min	Cardio 25 min Variable Stretch	Weights: Upper Body Abs Cardio 20	Free Movement Day 30min Stretch
Week 2	Weights: Lower Body Abs Cardio 15 min HIIT	Cardio 40 min Stretch	Weights: Upper Body (no arms) Abs HIIT 15 min	Cardio 30 min Variable Arms Stretch	Weights: Lower Body Abs Cardio 20 min	Cardio 30 min Chest Press and Flyes HIIT 8 min Stretch	Free Movement Day 30 movement minimum
Week 3	Cardio 40 min Rows Abs Stretch	Weights: Full Body HIIT 10	Cardio 40 min Abs Stretch	Weights: Lower Body Abs 20 min Cardio	Cardio 45 min Arms Stretch	Weights: Upper Body HIIT 15	Free Movement Day/Rest

Week 4	Weights: Lower Body	Lower Body	Weights: Upper Body	Cardio	Weights: Lower Body	Cardio	Full Body
	Abs	Cardio 30 min	Abs	60 min	HIIT 15	30 min	Abs HIIT 18 min HIIT
	Cardio	Stretch	HIIT 10 min	Abs	Abs		
	40 min			Stretch			Celebrate!!!

Please refer to Appendix for Exercise Journals

My Living Sexy Fit Commitment

I am committed to the Living Sexy Fit Lifestyle Challenge beginning today.

I am doing this for myself because I understand that this transformation begins with me. I care about myself enough to let go of old patterns and behaviors that no longer serve me.

My past failures do not define me. Today, with my self-knowledge and willingness to change, I am prepared to embrace my inner confidence, strength, and positive self-image full on.

I realize this is work and accept the self-care price I must pay to achieve my mental and physical transformation. I will expect and adapt to adversity and embrace tough times as learning opportunities.

I will strive to take action and not to ruminate, bitch, moan, or whine. I commit to pursuing progress, not perfection, in my eating and training.

I will find joy to neutralize my stress and strive to become a master regrouper. I will be self-assertive and fight for the right to take care of myself. I will acknowledge and reward myself for my achievements along the way.

By completing the Challenge, I signify honor and respect for myself and affirm that I deserve health, happiness, and joy. To this end, I make the following commitments to myself over the following 28 days.

1.

2.

3.

I am 100% committed to the highest and best version of me.

Sincerely,

Your Signature _____

Printed Name _____

Please feel free to e-mail a copy of this to the LSF Accountability Team at the following address:
accountability@kate-mckay.com

"Celebrate each and every success you experience.

Don't wait for someone else to celebrate for you."
"Let the celebration come from within!"

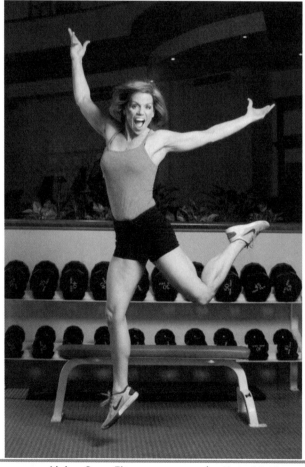

FAQs

"How long will it take to see results?"

When you begin to follow the LSF Lifestyle of eating clean and exercise, you will find almost immediately that you have increased energy and a healthy glow. As for weight loss, if that is your goal, each person will experience a different rate due to variations such as overall health, genetics, amount of exercise output, and commitment to eating clean.

Plan on losing 1½ to 2 lbs. per week on average, with some weeks more than others.

"I don't think I can eat this much food!"

I get it! But trust me, when you are eating the LSF Clean Eats way, you will be shocked how your body burns and churns all the yummy fuel. Your energy will be more consistent, and your vibrancy will go through the roof. Count on it!

Feel free, if you are not totally famished after 2½ to 3 hours, to make the next meal slightly smaller – but whatever you do, please don't skip! Your metabolism will go on slo-mo!

"How can I avoid midlife weight gain muffin top?

- Eat breakfast.
- Exercise regularly, doing both cardio and weights.
- Eat enough protein.
- Get a good night's sleep.

- Avoid alcohol.
- Drink lots of water.
- Limit stress.

"Cripes, Kate. You eat all the time. How come??"

The ticket to being Sexy Fit is to embrace grazing. Studies show that eating more frequently each day keeps the metabolism elevated; as a result, you will burn more calories throughout the day. Choose healthy lean proteins and vegetables as your primary meal sources, and eat moderate amounts of fruit and healthy fats to keep you going.

"Should I eat before I work out?"

Absolutely! To perform optimally, fuel your muscles in the hour before hitting the gym with a 150- to 250-calorie snack. Try a rice cake with a tablespoon of natural peanut butter, or a half cup of lowfat cottage cheese with 6 to 12 almonds, or a Granny Smith apple with a tablespoon of almond butter. A double chocolate doughnut is not considered a healthy snack! The body needs fuel to perform at its best. Make the most of your workout by starting with a full tank. You will be glad you did.

"What is DOMS?"

DOMS stands for delayed-onset muscle soreness, or what I call the "36-hour rule." After a vigorous workout, your muscles have depleted their glycogen store. Also during your workout, your muscles experience micro-trauma to the muscle fibers. As a result, muscle soreness ensues. How sore you are depends on the intensity and duration of your workout, your hormone levels, and how well your tank is fueled. It is imperative that, after completing a vigorous workout, you hydrate, eat healthy, and rest to allow the body to recover. Maximize your benefits by giving the body what it needs for restoration. Make your restoration time as important as your workouts. Some may call it extreme self-care. I call it smart living!

"What's all the buzz about yoga?"

Yoga is thousands of years old but is still a new concept for many of us. There are many different practices of yoga, so if you are interested taking a class, be sure that you ask what method of yoga is taught and what the teacher's credentials are. Make the teacher aware of your injuries or limitations so she can offer posture modifications. Start slowly and be gentle with yourself. A flexible body is a strong body, and yoga is a wonderful way to increase your flexibility, thereby reducing your chance of injury. Yoga is also great for increasing body awareness, reducing stress, and connecting the mind and the body. Studies show that you can achieve greater results in your workouts through visualization of specific muscles. This mind/body connection will improve your workouts and benefit other phases of your life. I believe that by connecting to the body, great things can happen. Celebrate your body through movement whether it is yoga, weight training, walking your dog, or skipping with your kids to the bus stop. Reclaim your freedom of movement. Don't use age, injury, lack of time, or whatever other tape runs through your mind as an excuse any longer. You have nothing to lose and a whole lot to gain. Make it a great day!

"Will I look like a man? I won't get too big, will I? I don't want to get bulky!"

Over the past 20 years, I have been weight training, I have heard those questions and statements over and over again. And the answer is a resounding NO!

Research has shown over and over that women who engage in a regular strength training program enjoy a long list of healthy benefits. As you realize the advantages of strength training and start feeling the effects of increased vitality, your doubts and fears of "bulking up" will rapidly fade.

"I did it! I completed my 28 Day Plan. I am so excited about my progress. Now what?"

Congratulations! You stuck with it, created the vision and went for it. You must feel so proud of yourself. Bravo!

Now, keep going! Set new goals for yourself and go after them with passion. You deserve to live a rich and juicy life. And we celebrate this living sexy fit lifestyle, by taking it one micro-step at a time, and enjoying each and every success. The journey is not always easy, but it is worth it. And so are you.

ABOUT KATE MCKAY©

Kate McKay, LLC was founded in 2012 by Kate McKay, who is known as the "Master Motivator." The Company is headquartered in Newburyport, MA, a suburb of Boston.

Kate is a transformational speaker, coach, fitness guru, entrepreneur and mother whose passion is to spread her message of living a life of prosperity, health, and abundance. She coaches and consults clients to propel themselves forward and live a full-on, juicy life.

Aside from her book *Living Sexy Fit*, Kate has also recently released 3 e-books, as well as an online program *28-Day Living Fabulously Fit, From the Inside Out with Kate Mckay!* Kate also has recently completed her extensive coaching program, which helps her clients monetize what they love. Kate's second book, *Living Sexy Rich*, will be released in the late fall 2014.

Kate has a passion for fitness and inspires others to live their best life. In 2013, she competed in 3 National Fitness Bikini Competitions and placed in the top three of each show at the age of 50.

Prior to establishing Kate McKay, LLC, Kate founded and built a multi-million dollar business called Gold Siena/Gold Party New England, a precious metal dealer, which partners with people to build their own businesses, and to celebrate prosperity, financial freedom and abundant living in both business and in all areas of your life.

Kate motivates people who are passionate to want more in their life by showing them how to embrace their own sense of prosperity so they can live in their personal power. Her company focuses on the four B's of Prosperous Living: Beliefs, Body, Business and Bucks, which allows people to finally live their biggest, boldest and wildest dreams.

Kate McKay, LLC offers a suite of e-learning products including e-books, audios and other online courses in addition to live events, workshops and coaching programs. Kate speaks at leadership conferences, networking meetings and women's conferences world-wide.

REFERENCES

ACE Personal Trainer Manual American Council on Exercise, Third Edition, 2003.

Labrada, Lee – *The Lean Body Promise*. New York: HarperCollins Publishers, 2005.

Verstegen, Mark, and Williams, Pete. *Core Performance: The Revolutionary Workout Program to Transform Your Body and Your Life*. New York: Rodale Press, 2004.

LIST OF RECOMMENDED READING

Carr, Kris. *Crazy Sexy Diet.* Guilford, CT: Globe Pequot Press, 2011.

Greenwood-Robinson, Maggie. *The Biggest Loser Fitness Program with Maggie Greenwood-Robinson, PhD.* New York: Rodale, Inc., 2007.

Hyman M.D., Mark *The Blood Sugar Solution 10-Day Detox Diet.* New York: Little, Brown and Company, 2014.

Ida, Wendy. *Take Back Your Life.* Concord, NC: Comfort Publishing, LLC, 2012.

Labrada, Lee. *The Lean Body Promise.* New York: HarperCollins Publishers, 2005.

Rath, Tom. *Strengths Finder 2.0.* New York: Gallup Press, 2007.

Reno, Tosca. *The Eat-Clean Diet Recharged!* Mississauga, ON: Robert Kennedy Publishing, 2009.

Verstegen, Mark. *Core Performance: The Revolutionary Workout Program to Transform Your Body and Your Life.* New York: Rodale Press, 2004.

APPENDIX

- My Living Sexy Fit Commitment
- Shopping List
- Meal Plan
- Exercise Journal – Upper Body
- Exercise Journal – Lower Body
- Exercise Journal – Stretching

My Living Sexy Fit Commitment

I am committed to the Living Sexy Fit Lifestyle Challenge beginning today.

I am doing this for myself because I understand that this transformation begins with me. I care about myself enough to let go of old patterns and behaviors that no longer serve me.

My past failures do not define me. Today with my self-knowledge and willingness to change, I am prepared to embrace my inner confidence, strength, and positive self-image full on.

I realize this is work and accept the self-care price I must pay to achieve my mental and physical transformation. I will expect and adapt to adversity and embrace tough times as learning opportunities.

I will strive to take action and not to ruminate, bitch, moan, or whine. I commit to pursuing progress, not perfection, in my eating and training.

I will find joy to neutralize my stress and strive to become a master re-grouper. I will be self-assertive and fight for the right to take care of myself. I will acknowledge and reward myself for my achievements along the way.

By completing the Challenge, I signify honor and respect for myself and affirm that I deserve health, happiness, and joy.

To this end, I make the following commitments to myself over the following 28 days.

      1.
      2.
      3.
I am 100% committed to the highest and best version of me.

Sincerely,

Signature _____

Printed Name _____

Please feel free to email a copy of this to the LSF Accountability Team at the following address: accountability@kate-mckay.com

FOOD SHOPPING LIST

PROTEIN	NON-STARCHY VEGETABLES	STARCHY VEGETABLES	FRUIT	GOOD FAT
Lean beef cuts	Lettuce	Oatmeal	Grapefruit	Almond oil
Chicken breast	Broccoli	Brown rice	Blueberries	Olive oil
Turkey breast	Zucchini	Rice cakes	Strawberries	Flaxseed oil
Ground turkey	Cauliflower	Spaghetti squash	Raspberries	Fish/tuna oil
Eggs/egg whites	Spinach	Sweet potatoes	Blackberries	Almonds
Haddock	Green beans	Ezekiel bread	Apples	Cashews
Cod	Asparagus	Whole grain pasta	Pears	Walnuts
Halibut	Peppers	Yams	Bananas	Salmon
Flounder	Kale	Pumpkin		Avocados
Salmon	Onions	Quinoa		Coconut oil
Swordfish	Mushrooms			Walnut oil
Tuna				
Tofu				
Tempeh				
Protein Powder				

Living Sexy Fit   by Kate McKay

The Meal Plan

Date: **Day _____ of 28**

Total Protein   Total Protein

Total Carbs   Total Carbs

Total Fats   Total Fats

PLAN	ACTUAL

Meal 1   Meal 1

  a.m.   a.m.

  p.m.   p.m.

Meal 2   Meal 2

  a.m.   a.m.

  p.m.   p.m.

Living Sexy Fit   by Kate McKay

Meal 3	Meal 3
a.m.	a.m.
p.m.	p.m.
Meal 4	Meal 4
a.m.	a.m.
p.m.	p.m.
Meal 5	Meal 5
a.m.	a.m.
p.m.	p.m.
Meal 6	Meal 6
a.m.	a.m.
p.m.	p.m.

Exercise Journal – Upper Body

Date: Planned Start Time: Actual Start Time:

Day _____ of 28   Planned End Time: Actual End Time:

Upper Body Workout   Time to Complete: Total Time:

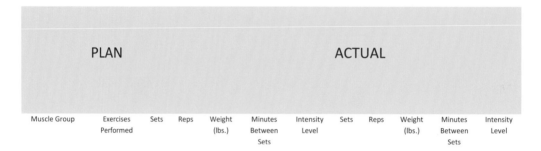

Muscle Group	Exercises Performed	Sets	Reps	Weight (lbs.)	Minutes Between Sets	Intensity Level	Sets	Reps	Weight (lbs.)	Minutes Between Sets	Intensity Level
			PLAN						ACTUAL		

Chest

Shoulders

Back

| Muscle Group | PLAN | | | | | | ACTUAL | | | | |
	Exercises Performed	Sets	Reps	Weight (lbs.)	Minutes Between Sets	Intensity Level	Sets	Reps	Weight (lbs.)	Minutes Between Sets	Intensity Level
Triceps											
Biceps											
Cardio											

Exercise Journal – Lower Body

Date: Planned Start Time: Actual Start Time:

Day _____ of 28   Planned End Time: Actual End Time:

Lower Body Workout   Time to Complete: Total Time:

	PLAN						ACTUAL				
Muscle Group	Exercises Performed	Sets	Reps	Weight (lbs.)	Minutes Between Sets	Intensity Level	Sets	Reps	Weight (lbs.)	Minutes Between Sets	Intensity Level
Quadriceps & Hamstrings											
Calves											

Exercise Journal – Stretch Series

Date: Planned Start Time: Actual Start Time:

Day _____ of 28   Planned End Time: Actual End Time:

Stretch Series   Time to Complete: Total Time:

		PLAN						ACTUAL			
Muscle Group	Exercises Performed	Sets	Reps	Weight (lbs.)	Minutes Between Sets	Intensity Level	Sets	Reps	Weight (lbs.)	Minutes Between Sets	Intensity Level

Shoulders

Chest

Sides

	PLAN						ACTUAL				
Muscle Group	Exercises Performed	Sets	Reps	Weight (lbs.)	Minutes Between Sets	Intensity Level	Sets	Reps	Weight (lbs.)	Minutes Between Sets	Intensity Level

Hips

Thighs

Hamstrings

Living Sexy Fit   by Kate McKay

Living Sexy Fit by Kate McKay

www.LivingSexyFit.com